LIFE **BEYOND**
HEADACHES

Dr. Jeffry Finnigan

LIFE BEYOND HEADACHES

Published by:
Finnigan Clinic
1307 Violet S.E.
Olympia, WA 98503

SECOND EDITION
Published by the Finnigan Clinic
1307 Violet S.E.
Olympia, WA 98503

The cartoon in Chapter Nine is printed with permission from John McPherson.

The various clip art were taken from ©1995 Softkey International, Inc., and its licensors.

The artwork on pages 98, 109,. 115 & 118, were taken, with permission, from the booklet, *Atlas Orthogonal Chiropractic*, Vogel Enterprises, Inc., 1982
15300 Ten Mile Road, E. Detroit, MI 48021.
2nd Edition 1987, 3rd Edition 1990.

Table of Contents

Acknowledgments   vi
Dedication   vii
Introduction   viii
Preface   ix

Chapter: **Page:**

1 - Headaches ... They're for Real   1

2 - One Bone   11

3 - Life-force   18

4 - The BIG Idea   22

5 - Inductive and Deductive Reasoning   40

6 - **AIR** (Foundational Key #1)   ⚷— 50

7 - The Linch Pin Theory of Health
        and Disease   58

8 - **FOOD AND WATER**
        (Foundational Key #2)   ⚷— 67

9 - **EXERCISE** (Foundational Key #3)   ⚷— 89

10 - **SLEEP** (Foundational Key #4)   ⚷— 94

11 - **POSITIVE MENTAL
         ATTITUDE** (Foundational Key #5)   ⚷— 100

12 - **A HEALTHY NERVE SYSTEM**
         (Foundational Key #6)   ❁—⚷ 106

13 - Where the Rubber Meets the Road   113

         Foundational Key Action List   124

APPENDIX: Testimonials

THIS BOOK IS PRINTED IN SLIGHTLY LARGER FONT AND SPACED TO ENHANCE THE READING EXPERIENCE FOR THOSE SUFFERING WITH HEADACHES.

• Acknowledgments •

As I consider all the people who have contributed in one way or another to whom I would like to express my appreciation for their ideas, suggestions, and support in making this book a reality the list continues to grow. First, I would like to thank my wife and family for allowing me to be "different, and providing the environment to be creative." To my dear friend in Australia, Dr. Robert Cowin. The seeds of the *"big idea"* were first sown in me many years ago by Drs. Joseph Flesia and Guy Riekeman, whom I thank. Equally, Bill Esteb and Dr. Dick Benson are always ready with some insight and encouragement. Drs. Daniel Murphy, Dennis Harding, Fred Vogel, Erick Ohlsen, I thank you. Many thanks, also, to Gloria Fletcher, Robyn Marshall, Jane Fitzpatrick, and Karen Alexander. Finally, thank you to Jay Gigandet for your artistic suggestions.

• Dedication •

To Roy W. Sweat, D.C.

Who gave me my start in the upper cervical discipine. Who showed an interest in me at an early age by gently, yet firmly, guiding me to strive for excellence, and for grand results. He's my friend, my brother, and my mentor. He's a guy who remembers a good joke when he hears one. He's someone who'll be there when the chips are down, yet he focuses on the good in any situation.

• Introduction •

Rather than another self help book, I hope that this will prove to be a self actualization catalyst. It is my sincere wish that by reading this book we accomplish three things. First, that the information contained herein will allow you to <u>understand</u> that if you have chronic headaches there is hope. Second, the information contained in this book will actually help you rid yourself of ongoing chronic headache pain and regain your normal lifestyle. And third, serve as a launching pad to a new personal philosophy about the simplicity of health and your body. Let's start by providing you an interesting perspective on your body, your life, and your headaches.

• Preface •

- If you have less energy than you think you should.
- If you have what aspirin manufacturers refer to as "ordinary everyday headaches."
- If you are frustrated with the lack of real answers from your doctor(s).
- If you're fed up with impersonal and ineffective health care.
- If you are ready to deal with causes, rather than just treating symptoms.
- If you are concerned that the pills you're being told to swallow may be more harmful than your original headaches.
- If your <u>bathroom</u> cabinet has turned into a <u>medicine</u> cabinet.
- If you're just plain sick and tired of being sick and tired.
- And finally ... If you're ready to reclaim responsibility for your life and health, if someone would just make sense of it all, and provide a little guidance.

Then welcome to the re-discovery of your vital "Life-force."

I know that you know you have this power within you. But through the years of clever pharmaceutical marketing, domineering medical institutions, and invasive procedures, we have all but forgotten that the only healing power resides within us. As the late Robert Mendelsohn M.D. once stated, "It's O.K. to talk about this healing power within on Sunday, but Monday through Saturday we are expected to put our faith in the *church of modern medicine.*" The only predictable healing that can occur is when the doctor and the patient realize together that the patient has a health problem, but the patient also brings the actual healing mechanism along within.

Your healing mechanism might be broken down right now, you may have forgotten that you have it, or it may just be asleep. Therefore, I'll do my best to re-awaken and re-introduce you to that which you may faintly realize you actually possess. The most magnificent power to tune into and access, is your inborn Life-force which flows throughout your body.

In reading this book, I promise to help you feel better about yourself and your health decisions, whatever they may be. I will give you the data for the six foundational keys to health amplification.

Think for a moment about the term *health amplification.* In order to amplify something one must assume that he or she already possess that "thing" (in this case health). Would you like your health amplified?

Of course! Who wouldn't? Now, if you answered yes, then you must agree that you have at least some health within. So let's figure out if we can turn up the volume. Let's talk about amplifying your health! I know how to do that, and I can teach you if you're willing to play. So, are you?

By the way, most people are somewhat ignorant (that's not

derogatory) about the concept of health amplification. With the knowledge you're about to gain, you will not only begin the process of eliminating your headaches, but also be able to make pivotal decisions in your life from a position of understanding and power, rather than ignorance and submission. Isn't that nice? Plus, we'll make it fun, keep it simple, and entertaining.

Before we end this short preface, I want to remind you that the number one starting point for our trip together (and I know you already knew this)...... is that health and healing is an inside job. The human body has everything it needs. No doctor has ever grown new heart cells, blood, or bone tissue for his or her patient. But your body is doing it for you every day! Health always comes from within, and I don't mean you put a pill inside and you begin healing! The "within" I'm talking about is deeper ... much deeper.

Let's validate your reasons for reading this book. First, I want you to know that I know that there truely can be ......

LIFE BEYOND
HEADACHES

• Chapter One •

HEADACHES ... THEY'RE FOR REAL

A doctor can't do a biopsy on your brain and find the head-ache. Blood tests, urine analysis, CT scans, and every other medical test you can name do not demonstrate a patient's head-ache objectively. The headache usually is an end in itself. There's no fractured bone, or ulcer to objectively see. Therein lies some of the initial problem with communicating your pain to others. Your family and friends sympathize, for the most part, but after a while they may make you feel a little uncomfortable when, once again, you're not up to par. You try to explain to them, but there is nothing to show them. And if they've never really experienced chronic headaches them-selves, they don't get it. Up until now, "pain" was all we've had ... no other hard facts. It's all been rather subjective.

But headaches are a real syndrome, a serious condition that is costing our nation billions of dollars in treatment costs and time loss. More important, it's costing many the quality of their lives. Chronic headaches can virtually destroy fami-lies and relationships.

MEDICINE MISDIRECTED

Medical doctors are some of the hardest-working, most sin-cere individuals I have met. They've invested several hundred thousand dollars into their education, sacrificed family time, and they keep late hours for those "on call" weekends. But, so much of medical attention is spent on treating *symptoms* and most doctors rarely think in terms of correcting or dealing with *causes*. As a society, we have just recently begun to think more in terms of long-term consequences and prevention. So, it's no surprise that when a patient shows up at the hospital to remove a cancerous lung, we hope and pray for the best outcome. But what about the last 20 years of a "pack a day"? The medical doctors' hands are tied. Their situation is much like a mechanic, ready to fix the breakdown after the damage is done.

Do you know anyone who takes their kids to the doctor for antibiotics at the first sign of the sniffles? Is that prevention? Only if you consider robbing the child of the opportunity to naturally experience micro organisms and build his or her own strong immune response mechanisms. You can't kill all the "bugs" on the planet. We and our children need to adapt to the environment. Again, the doctors' hands are tied. The parent comes in with the condition already diagnosed, and demands the "appropriate" dosage of the latest pharmacopoeia. The doctor needs to satisfy and calm the parent, so generally the doctor complies. Unfortunately, this process contributes to a super breed of microbes, as the drug never kills all the microbes, just the weak ones, leaving the drug - resistant "bugs" alive to reproduce. Therefore, the child's immune system is hampered. Unfortunately, the doctor's decision to treat the symptoms rather than correct the cause contributes to a growing pool of antibiotic- resistant bacteria.

Regarding the treatment of symptoms, between $500 million

and $1billion per year is spent for over - the- counter head-ache medications alone. Do those medications correct the cause of the problem or do they just treat the symptoms? The total bill for headache pain alone per year in the U.S. in-cluding medication, time loss, and treatment of this national disaster, is upwards of $8 billion!

I want to strongly suggest to you that the same level of think-ing that got you where you are today, will definitely not get you where you want to go. The same mind set and same actions will only continue a problem. Albert Einstein is quoted as saying, "*to continue to do the same things, and to expect a new result, now that's insanity.*" If your present and past treatments have not been providing a real solution to your problem, then perhaps you're ready for a new ap-proach. To begin the process to an improved life, you need to gain new data. New information will allow you to choose a new approach to an old problem. Initially, you will be the only beneficiary. But, in time, those you spend time with, your family members (children and grandchildren) and friends, will feel the impact of your enhanced life. Take a moment and think of others who will benefit as you regain control of your life.

It is in this spirit that I hope you will find this book useful. My attempt is to give you a fresh perspective and a new direction. Let's not just treat symptoms, control pain or manage lives around the headaches; let's find out how to amplify wellness and discover the actual cause of headaches. Then, let's use non-invasive technology to allow your body to correct, balance and prevent the damn things from returning! If that sounds exciting, you'll be happy to know that ...

CHRONIC HEADACHES... NOT JUST IN YOUR HEAD

During the past 20 years of my work with headache patients, a few points stand out that are worth mentioning in the beginning. First, most of these people have suffered from headaches for months and sometimes years. They have, to some extent, learned to "deal with it." Dealing with it means different things to different people. To some, it might mean spending two or three hours in the middle of an otherwise busy day secluded in a dark room. To others, dealing with chronic headache means never leaving home without a supply of medications, from aspirin to prescription pain killers.

Nearly all who suffer from chronic headache admit that this condition has cost them dearly in their personal lives.....divorces, loss of income, strained relationships with family members and friends. Approximately 65 percent of these chronic headache cases (clinically observed at our facilities) are female, which is a significant number. But those statistics also indicate that men comprise a substantial 35 percent. Also noteworthy is the public's general concept that headache is not really an authentic health disorder. It is a troublesome misconception that chronic headache is a condition easily swept aside by popping a couple of pills and going on one's way. Your spouse (or even a doctor) who has never experienced this pain can find it difficult to believe that your condition is real. But when the throbbing doesn't leave, and you can't explain that you are all but incapacitated by this "fictitious" condition, it is extremely frustrating, to say the least. In addition to the actual pain, a person can also experience feelings of guilt and despair because he or she can't fully navigate through the day. This condition that is considered trivial by those who don't experience the relentless pain is increasingly frustrating due to its intangible nature.

The fact that headaches can't be identified and removed, like a tumor or an ulcer that can be detected on X-ray, does not make it any less a real disorder. Drug addiction and alcoholism can't be X-rayed, yet they are very real problems. I contend that chronic headache is a genuine physiological (not psychological) disorder that needs to be taken seriously. I believe it is as real a disorder as heart disease or cancer. And although one might not die directly as a natural result of the condition itself (as with cancer), a number of the chronic headache patients I've consulted with have seriously pondered a way out of their body. The second edition of *Clinically Oriented Anatomy*, by Keith Moore, describes how in certain types of aggravated neck conditions the ganglion of the second cervical nerve can be compressed between the top two vertebrae. "This may result in prolonged headaches in the occipital region so severe that they may result in suicidal tendencies," he wrote. In writing this book I want to provide you with hope, based on fact, and to create a bond with you. I also hope that we can be thankful that your headache episodes have never been so bad that you considered suicide, but if they have... you are now realizing that there is a way out.

One reference by F. Sheftell and A. Rapoport, stated that headache is a real disorder (I agree), but described it as a biological condition, for which there is no cure at the present time. These authors suggest that headache could only be controlled (I presume by chemicals) but not corrected. I totally disagree... because in my experience the overwhelming majority of chronic headache conditions are primarily caused by structure. Individual headache episodes are often "triggered," secondarily, by a number of considerations including biological triggers. But clinical evidence demonstrates that when *particular structural elements* (to be described) *are in balance it is very difficult to get a headache.* Also, we will share insight from mainstream medical literature that validates exactly what I am proposing. Therefore, CHRONIC HEADACHES CAN BE CURED, NOT JUST TREATED.

You know what headaches are and what they feel like, but we need to define the word "chronic,"so that you'll know if your experience fits into the context of this book. The word chronic is defined by Webster's dictionary as ... "Lasting a long time or recurring often. Also, by habit, custom, or ritual... habitual." So if you've suffered with headaches for more than six months (a time period I've chosen-you may have suffered for decades), and if they recur often, almost habitually, let's say 2-3 times per month (although you may have them more frequently, even constantly) then I think you will benefit from reading this book. So the term "chronic" defined for our purpose is a period of six months or more and recurring frequently.

WHY YOU'RE STILL LOOKING FOR RESULTS

If you're like most people with headaches you've tried a lot of medications and over- the- counter pain killers. That's certainly a reasonable short-term solution to controlling one's pain. But over time the body's ability to produce its own natural endorphins (pain killers) becomes hampered. That's exactly why you may find yourself taking larger and larger doses of medication. The drugs become less effective and you have to take more pills to achieve the same relief. Additional side effects from ingesting these chemicals include depression, fatigue, and digestive disorders, and often times the pill you're taking <u>for</u> headache pain can actually <u>cause more headaches</u>! Commonly called rebound headaches.

The answer to correcting your problem is not going to be found in a pill bottle. This reminds me a little bit of the obese person who is looking for the magic diet pill that will remove all of those undesirable pounds. Pills didn't put the weight on and pills won't take the weight off, at least not permanently. The same is true of headaches.

The power to cure your headache for good is within. Except for the extremely rare brain tumor or some other exotic situation that occurs in less than one percent of all headache sufferers, you will not need surgery, injections, or harmful medications. What you will need is to reestablish your internal balance, releasing the flow of your Life-force from above, down and inside out. If the preceding sounds a bit too philosophical for you, hang on- the technology exists to accomplish precisely what we're talking about.

THE TRUTH ABOUT HEADACHE CAUSES

Most people who have lived extended periods of time with headaches have believed, at one time or another, that they have a brain tumor, a blood disorder or cancer. Certainly there are exotic causes for chronic headaches including the ones I just mentioned. But those are rare and can be ruled out with proper medical tests.   If you've come this far with chronic headaches, your doctor has probably already run those tests.

IT'S ALL IN YOUR HEAD!

"Well of course it is ... at least the pain seems to be. That's why they're called <u>head</u>-aches!" *But* the brain itself cannot feel pain. You could actually touch parts of the brain and you wouldn't feel it. Surgeries that are performed on the brain are sometimes done under a local anesthesia. The brain is exposed, and the surgeon is looking right at it and touching it, while the patient is awake and alert.

On the inside, the brain is floating in a liquid bath called cerebral spinal fluid. Just as the pregnant mother provides her unborn fetus embryonic fluid in the womb to float in for protection, the brain is encased inside the skull and floats in its own fluid for the very same reason. The brain itself is the consistency of gelatin, or that of cooked spaghetti, and is very delicate. For further protection, a tissue called meninges covers the entire brain and spinal cord. Think of this tissue as a nylon stocking blanketing the contour of a woman's leg. If a person was unfortunate enough to have a brain tumor, the pain he or she might feel (in the way of headache) would likely be from pressure and resultant deformation of the meninges; it has pain sensation capabilities unlike the brain. This type of headache pain would be considered internal, or intracranial pain and, as mentioned, is extremely rare.

The nerves, muscles around the skull, and blood vessels all have sensory input capabilities. "Sensory input" means that the tissues have the ability to transmit pain signals to the brain. These tissues and their relationship to surrounding structure is most likely the cause of 99% of all headaches. These are considered extracranial headaches. Amazingly, these tissues can cause extreme pain perceived by the victim as being inside the brain (you might swear that someone has a drill *inside* your head). Also, nausea, dizziness, fatigue, impaired vision, even depression can arise from extracranial headache. Although this type of headache is not life threatening, it certainly has destroyed the quality of life for millions.

Another concern people often have is that they may have a personality that produces headaches. One might feel they over-react to situations during the day causing "stress" headaches. Headaches are *not caused* by your mind, your stress level, or your diet. However, these factors can look like they are the very cause, simply because they are actually the triggers for headaches in most people. **Read carefully now**. I said those events will *trigger headaches, but they are not the cause*. Women who have headaches for two or three days the same time each month, certainly have good reason to believe that hormones can cause headaches. I would agree that personality, stress, hormones and other factors definitely play a contributing role in the continual production of this frustrating condition. But clinical evidence demonstrates that these factors do not cause the headaches. I've had people tell me they've been diagnosed as having a "migraine personality." I've never met a migraine personality, nor does literature support such a concept. These factors that we've mentioned: hormones, personality and diet (we'll discuss later), are simply contributing factors, they are triggers. If there is live ammunition in the firing chamber, and you pull one of those triggers, chances are you'll set off another headache. <u>The "cause" was already in place</u>.

The questions that need to be asked are: If hormones, stress, and diet are just triggers for setting off the headache ... what is the live ammunition? Why is it that someone can have a stressful day and be out of commission with head pain for two or three days, yet that same person endures the same type of stress- filled day two weeks later, and does not get a headache? How is it that a woman will start her menstrual cycle ... but the real cause of headache is not present on a particular month ... so no headache? It's wonderful for these people when this happens ... now, how can we make it happen more often?

What is the overwhelming "common" cause of 90+ percent of all headaches? Our clinical experience demonstrates a common link between the patient with "stress headaches" and the patient with "menstrual headaches." The patient with "migraines" has this in common with the patient who suffers from "cluster headaches." That common denominator is ......

• Chapter Two •

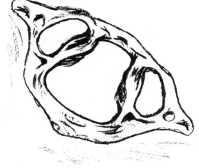

ONE BONE

"Well done is better than well said."
--Benjamin Franklin

Linda presented herself at my office on a wet Western Washington spring day. She arrived tired and slightly gaunt after a full day of "on- the- job" data entry.

After Linda filled out the short entrance form, my staff showed her back to the examination room, offered her a cup of tea, which she accepted, and told her that Dr. Finnigan would be along in a short while.

When I looked over the Patient Information Form she had just filled out, I began to understand why she had told my staff that I was her last hope. My form inquires about Headaches, Insomnia, Muscle pain, Neck and Back pain, Depression, Low Energy, and on and on. Linda had checked virtually every one of the 25 or 30 symptoms we had listed in the affirmative, indicating she was living within a "tidal wave" of ill health.

I asked Linda how long she had been dealing with all of these health problems. She reported that she'd been a healthy, happy mother of two until she'd taken a fall on a slick stair step, three years prior. At first she thought nothing of the fall, other than the embarrassment and a few bruises.

For a few days she felt fine, but developed a migraine type headache on the fourth day; though at the time she did not associate the headache with the fall. She had never had a migraine before. This initial headache lasted a day and a half, then cleared, but she was left feeling drained of energy. A couple of days passed, and from then on she would consistently have either an "eyeball" headache, as she described sharp pains behind her right eye, or she would have a full blown "sick" migraine headache. Linda's eyes were very sensitive to light, and she would almost always wear sunglasses. Within a year, other physical pains, chronic fatigue, insomnia, and depression had set in. By then, the only thing she could pin her persistent health problems on was her fall.

I asked Linda what she had done to treat these problems... that's when the tears began to flow. She belonged to a Health Maintenance Organization (HMO). Her doctor initially treated her with anti-inflammatory and headache medication. That didn't seem to help; in fact, in time the drugs aggravated her problems. Linda went back to her HMO doctors countless times over the next two years. During that time, she had been X-rayed, urine tested, blood tested, CAT scanned, MRI'd, and re-X-rayed. More tests were performed, and more medications prescribed for an inconclusive diagnosis. At one point Linda was even put on a broad spectrum antibiotic for some elusive mystery infection, all to no avail.

After a year and a half, she had spent personal funds and several days in a specialized Headache Clinic, and at a Pain Control Center. Linda had received some relief from acupuncture and had fair results from chiropractic care.

But as she put it, "the lack of energy, the lack of quality sleep and the continual throbbing pains were really driving me crazy."

Then she confided that she didn't really know why she was even at my office. "You're not a participating member of my HMO," she blurted, "and besides, I've already tried a chiropractic doctor. The only reason that I'm here is because my friend Sarah brought me here. She said you did something different for her husband that turned his problems around after his regular doctors couldn't help him. She said you have some sort of system that is different."

At that point I knew that Linda was open to a fresh approach for her problems. In that instant, I realized that although she was terribly frustrated....she still had hope, and with that hope was the seed of her willingness to try.

After a brief examination, I assured her that my approach would be completely opposite of the failed medical treatments that she had endured. I also informed her that it would not include any manipulation of her neck, which she said the two previous doctors had done with little benefit. I explained that just as there are many specialties within medicine, chiropractic is expanding its technological base also, and I felt that our system might just be right for her. I told her that my postgraduate studies have centered around one bone, the area at the very top of the spine, just below the skull. This is a critical area to have correctly balanced, due to the important vascular and neurological components associated with this region. It is not an easy area to balance properly. I've rarely seen it done through manipulation, and never through surgery.

I also informed her that her little fall could have easily caused a mal-position of that bone, which could, in turn, be the critical "missing link" in her recovery.

Linda's examination revealed that the "one bone" I had mentioned, the Atlas, was not synchronized with her skull, nor the rest of her body. It is the first cervical vertebrae and is structurally unlike any other area of the body. Linda's Atlas was compromising her nerves and blood vessels. She had a condition called Atlas Neuro Vascular Syndrome (ANVS), which requires a specific technology aided by patient compliance, in order to help her reach her goals.

But what I was about to say to Linda was going to be the turning point in my career. My words were not mine, they just came out unplanned. In reality, these words, happily, were the turning point of her life also.

She was a pleasant woman. She had suffered so long without any noticeable improvement. She had spent so much money with no lasting results. I did not want to contribute my name to her list of failures, nor did I want to add more to her economic woes. I felt so strongly that our Atlas technology was perfect for Linda, these unplanned words came spilling out of my mouth as if I had no control over what was being said. As I listened to what "I" was saying, I was nearly as shocked as she was.

I told Linda that I would accept her case and I would do my complete work-up on her so she could experience my technique and actually begin care to remove the cause of her problems. **And** ... If she didn't notice a significant and substantial improvement immediately, or within a short while, she could walk away with no obligation. I didn't want to contribute to her financial burden for something that was unproductive. I didn't want to join the failed medical system, and add more insult to her near emotional, spiritual, and physical collapse.

She was astonished at the opportunity I tendered. Her face lifted, her eyes brightened, it was obvious that she was instantly freed from the fear of failure. She had <u>nothing to lose</u> and everything to gain. She would participate completely. "I've never heard of a doctor doing that before," she said. Neither had I. Then, she asked, "Are you that confident in your work?"

To which I replied, "If I am right about your condition, and your problems are caused by neuro-vascular pressure at the Atlas area, then yes, I'm that confident that this might be the only way out of your fix. You and I will both know in a few short minutes if we are on the right track. Nothing else will relieve the problem if it is stemming from there. If I'm wrong, then you'll be no worse for the treatment. I won't want to waste any more of your money, nor my time." With Linda's smile I knew that my offer was more than fair.

I also informed her that in addition to utilizing my specialized technique, she would have the responsibility of making some small changes in her life. There were five other key components needed to amplify her health since she had been in this rut for three years.

Together, I call these the **Foundational Keys for Health Amplification**. In Linda's case, in addition to my specialized form of care, she must also **HELP** pull herself up and out by :

1) Breathing properly, to allow proper oxygenation of the cells of the body. This is necessary to step up the function of the whole body.
2) Eating appropriately, in a way that empowers her body, rather than just filling it.
3) Getting a modest amount of exercise.
4) Getting some real rest.
5) Reestablishing the positive mental attitude she had three years ago.

And, finally...

6) H.N.S. Maintaining a <u>Healthy Nerve System</u>.

Linda didn't have a prayer on God's green earth to become a functioning human being again until someone removed the pressure from her nervous system, at the brain stem level, right up near the base of her skull. And that is my specialty. I have trained 20 years preparing for frustrating, non-responding cases like these related to the Atlas. Incidentally, the Atlas is paramount for Foundational Key # 6. If the Atlas isn't balanced you're not going to have a healthy, properly functioning nerve system. A **Healthy Nerve System** is the *Master Key* to the other 5. You will learn more about the Atlas and your nerve system in chapters 12 and 13.

My job as Linda's "health coach" was to offer her something that hadn't been done by numerous health care providers and doctors. My ultimate goal was to reconnect her Life-force and help her reclaim her life.

Linda agreed. If I was willing to forego payment to actually begin treatment, letting HER decide, letting HER be the judge and jury whether I was providing any value worthy of her investment of time and capital, then she was committed to W.E.I.T. (what ever it takes) to get her desired results.

Linda responded perfectly. Together we balanced her Atlas area and removed pressure from vital nerves and blood vessels. This success was accomplished painlessly, without drugs or chemicals of any kind. She followed my recommendations. Today she is 90 percent headache free and her energy level is way up. Linda has repeatedly stated she's had her life given back to her!

As noted earlier, life and health come from deep within. As you know, one can "treat" headaches on the surface with pills, but you want to get to the core of the problem. In order to increase the quality and quantity of your wellness, you need to be able to tap into the source. To get the most from this book it is now time to introduce you to your very own incredible......

• Chapter Three •

LIFE-FORCE

"May the Force be with you."
----Luke Skywalker to Han Solo in Star Wars

"Life-force." That's an interesting term, isn't it? All things that are alive exhibit some form of "intelligent" force or power. The ability to ingest and digest food is a power that we share with all living creatures from the single celled amoeba to the gigantic blue whale.

Adaptability is a great example of the power of the Life-force. People who have the ability to adapt are vibrant ... they thrive. People who cannot adapt sometimes find it difficult to fit into new situations. If a person's health is low, one may not be able to adapt to micro-organisms in the environment ... they fall susceptible. Why does one person sitting at the table, eating the same food, breathing the same air as his family members, not get sick -- while seven other members of his family come down with a full blown case of the flu? Answer... He encountered the same flu bugs, but unlike his family, he adapted. His vibrant body neutralized the invading agents.

Another example of the Life-force is the reflex reaction away from pain. If you were to put your hand on a red hot burner while in the kitchen, you probably wouldn't pause and ponder the melting temperature of your skin. How would you react? Without a moments hesitation your hand would fly off the burner. Pain is a protective and adaptive mechanism. You might not think so, but pain is actually your friend. Your headache pain is actually a warning, or an alarm, alerting you to take corrective action. Your body wants to be well. It's trying to tell you. Yet Madison Avenue has taught you that head pain is to be medicated and swept under the rug. This is an $18 billion lie. That's how much per year is spent to convince you, and me, that when we have any ache or pain the right and moral thing to do is pop some medication, bending our consciousness. In reality these drugs and medications lessen our "aliveness" and our ability to adapt. The pain is nothing more than an alarm. Your body is saying "help me adapt." All of these activities rely on what I call their inborn Life-force.

Dr. Bartlet Joshua Palmer, the developer of chiropractic, in his 1949 classic *The Bigness of the Fellow Within*, referred to the Life-force as an impulse, "the tiny rivulet of force that emanates from the mind and flows over the nerves to the cells and stirs them into life. The magic power that transforms common food into living, loving, thinking clay."

The presence of your Life-force is what differentiates you and me from a corpse. The corpse, at one time, also had a Life-force which now has departed -- that is the only difference. The corpse has a brain and nerve system, it has a heart, lungs, kidneys ... all the parts are there. A rock on the ground outside your home never did have a Life-force- it never ingested food, it didn't adapt to it's environment, it was never repelled by pain.

When the Life-force is allowed to fully express itself through your body, you are alive and more able to adapt to your environment. When the Life-force is hampered, you are going to experience less health, you are less able to adapt and your body does not rebound or perform as well as it should. The end result is a condition or symptom (such as chronic headache), that "necessitates" your attention and often the attention of professionals.

You may not have realized this until now but the brain of a living person, or an animal, not only controls all of the life maintaining functions of the organs within the body, but the brain also apparently generates real power. The living brain is a dynamo, like a rechargeable battery. I'll continue to refer to this power that flows from the brain throughout the body as your "Life-force."

Many years ago, laboratory rabbits were the victims of a rather brutal experiment. The rabbits were operated on and had electrodes inserted into their brains. Connections to those electrodes were left exposed externally on top of the rabbits' skull. The scientists then hooked up a small radio to the exposed connections and, amazingly, these rabbit-powered radios worked! The scientist theorized that the rabbits, and for that matter all living animals, have an electric current emanating from the brain and nerve system. Unfortunately, if the radios were left "on" for any length of time, the power required to run the radios would suck the Life-force right out of the rabbits, and they would die prematurely. So what did the scientists do? They just plugged in more rabbits to the radios, and soon those rabbits would also die.

The preceding being true, we can assume that the presence of, and the quality of, your Life-force can to a large degree determine your recovery and/or the amount of health you'll enjoy.

The question must be asked, can the quantity and quality of the expression of your Life-force be hindered or diminished? Just take a look around you. Do you see yourself enjoying the same level of well-being as you did five or 10 years ago? Do you know anyone 10 or 15 years older than you who seems to have more wellness and vitality? Comparative age is mentioned right away so you don't have a chance to say that you're not as young as you used to be! <u>That's no excuse</u>.

Your Life-force can be diminished and, in my opinion, this unfortunate experience is one of the greatest yet silent robbers of life and health on the planet today! Fortunately, you're not walking around town getting hooked up to radios by electrodes protruding from your head. But perhaps some old injuries and incidents that have happened to you, and some of your current habits, have created a condition that "draws" the power <u>out</u> of your body- much slower than the rabbits, but power loss just the same. Can it be stopped and turned around? Can we reclaim and amplify our Life-force? Absolutely! ..... And that is precisely what you're learning to do.

Let's take a step back from your own pain and headaches for a moment. As I mentioned earlier, rather than just dealing with your headache symptoms we want to strike at the root, and expand your complete wellness. In order to make a lasting impression, you need to own .....

• Chapter Four •

THE BIG IDEA

*"Discovery is seeing what everybody else has seen,
and thinking what nobody else has thought."*
--Albert Szent-Gyorgi

"But what if a person gets AIDS, or cancer, what would you do then?" My new patient asks the question with a slightly cynical tone. She knew I only have my hands and my knowledge to offer as a "healer." These are things that aren't mysterious like the stealthy procedures we all expect in the high tech environment of the modern hospital.

"You haven't got the Big Idea yet, Martha. Let me explain to you again how it all works." And so it goes, again and again, with so many of my encounters. What I do and say to my patients innately seems right to them, but our society has turned so far away from trusting the natural process, that part of my job has become re-teaching what they already know inside. For many, that inner voice hasn't been listened to for a very long time.

"How about Asthma? Can you help migraine headaches? I'll have to live with my ulcers, right? I've got high blood pressure so I'm to take these pills the rest of my life, but other than that I'm perfectly healthy."

I always try to put myself in my patients' shoes; I want to understand their concerns. Certainly, empathy is expected of a good and effective doctor. But, oh, how I wish you could sit on my side of the desk to hear and see the things that I hear and see.

So many people are missing the Big Idea in life and health. We (as a society) are so hung up on waiting for and treating our symptoms and our diseases that we've forgotten what health *really* is. If a person has cancer and he is magically "cured" of it, I know he would be extremely grateful, but I have a question. Now that the "tumor" is gone, is he truly healthy? Just because the end result of a disease is erased doesn't preclude the original cause of the problem. If the cause isn't dealt with, isn't it reasonable to think that the same process will continue? And in five years would he have another tumor? Treating the symptoms of disease is like pulling the head off a weed in your garden. If the root remains, in time you'll have another weed. One could name any other malady, replace the word cancer with the problem that you are dealing with right now such as headaches, and if your symptoms related to this condition "magically" vanished, instantly (I agree, anyone would want that to happen), but would you truly be healthy? I know you'd be happy, but are we interested in just removing the symptoms? If the person's condition magically disappeared, but the cause of the malfunction was left intact, then isn't it reasonable to assume that in time he or she would experience the same or worse situation? Treating painful symptoms is a necessary and important function of all doctors, but let's take an additional tack. With the obvious desire to feel more comfortable, we must also strike at the root of the problem and make the commitment to amplify our vitality, our immune system effectiveness and our reserves for wellness. Let's not forget that wellness is an option.

Part of this process will include a challenge to some of your present beliefs. I know some of you are swallowing prescription drugs. Few people admit that they do, but someone must be. The drug companies are far too wealthy not to have millions of folks buying their pills. Please read the remainder of this paragraph very attentively. **All** medications have side effects. That's not an inflammatory statement, I'm repeating what every pharmaceutical company knows. "All drugs have side effects" is another way of saying that drugs don't just influence their target organ. Let's go one step further ... If a healthy person were to take a prescription drug and continued for a period of time, that drug would eventually make a healthy body sick ... So, if that drug is going to make a healthy body ill ... *how on God's green earth could it possibly make a sick person well?* Interesting question, isn't it? Read that last paragraph over again if you are only skimming through this book.

So what exactly IS health? You and I want better health. If one really wants to attain a "state of being" or "an experience," to improve our chances of attaining our goal -- which is "health," we can vastly improve our chances of reaching that goal if we can identify, precisely describe, and visualize what we are going after. Chasing this goal is no different from chasing any other. Goal setting is imperative for your success. You must be able to see your goal in your "mind's eye." Imagine playing a game of basketball with no hoops. You would be confused. You'd be without any specific direction. Perhaps you might have a good time, but you really would be spinning your wheels. You couldn't keep score. And, in the case of our goal, I think few people have given much thought to what real health actually is. We tend not to think about our bodies unless ...what? That's right, we only think about them when they're NOT working. We end up thinking Health has something to do with our malfunctioning bodies! Health is not just the absence of pain!

Here is a word of caution: *Be careful of what you wish for, you might just get it!* Far wiser to have as a goal a state of wellness and optimum health (as a natural side effect ones pain would diminish), rather than shallowly wishing for a life without headaches. Many ill people live without having headaches, but you want more than that, I'm sure. Don't get caught lowering your expectations from life to meet your current situation. Raise your expectations, and change your situation! Other people enjoy health and happiness- why not you?

Since we've apparently forgotten what health really is, let's find a nice dry definition of <u>exactly</u> what "health" is. We'll start with a dictionary definition so there will be no contro-versy, at least over this portion of the book. Paraphrased *Dorland's Medical Dictionary* tells us that: HEALTH is a state of wholeness, in which all of the parts are functioning at 100%, all of the time. Now that's a pretty boring, unimpres-sive definition, wouldn't you agree? But look at it again- there are some critically important phrases. A state of wholeness, (so it's best if we're not missing parts) that's **functioning** at 100%. There's not much you and I can do about *time*. "Time," as one author put it, "is merciless." I'm totally convinced that the key to this formula, the one element that you and I can impact in our life experience, is **function**. All other aspects of the formula are set in stone, but function is the one variable. The liver FUNCTIONS differently under varying circumstances. The kidneys FUNCTION differently at times. All the cells of our bodies are designed to adapt and react at different rates of metabolism depending on what stresses are being imposed upon our bodies. Remember we talked about the people who did not develop headaches on particular occasions even though they had a stressful day, or were beginning a menstrual cycle? These were people who would normally get a headache under those circumstances. How well one's body is functioning at a particular time determines, by a far greater degree, how one will be feeling and performing. External stress and even hormonal changes pale when compared to the prime mover of function in the body.

So what controls the function of all the systems and cells of the body? What is the prime connector between your Lifeforce and a fully FUNCTIONING alive body?

Let's look to another respected medical textbook, *Gray's Anatomy*. This legendary text book tells us where health and healing come from. It tells us that the purpose of the brain and spinal cord is to control and regulate the function of all the tissues, organs, and systems, and to adapt the organism (you) to the environment. WOW! Now that's pretty important to know! If your goal is to become more healthy, we must agree that the preceding datum is *pivotal*.

There is no doubt that this bit of information and the pursuit of health from the "inside-out," represents a major difference from how the rest of the *civilized* world views health, from the "outside-in" (treatment with pills or potions from outside my body fix what is wrong inside). This serves to explain the results expected in an individual's life. Gray's tells us that we've got to have the nerve system flowing from above, down, and inside out for optimum function. This is your connector to your Life-force.

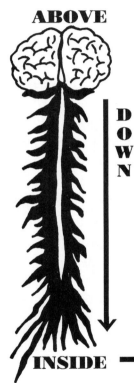

Many of my colleagues have an acronym "ADIO," which stands for ABOVE, DOWN, INSIDE OUT. All neurological functions and healing of the body, when you think about it, come from above, down and from the inside out. When little Johnny skins his knee we put an antiseptic and a bandaid on the wound. But does the healing come from the antiseptic and the bandaid? <u>No</u>. Would the scratches heal without the antiseptic and the bandaid? Certainly. So where does the healing power and the actual healing activity come from?

The body always heals itself from above, down, and inside out.

Healing comes from within (from the brain, down the spinal cord, and out to the periphery) from above, down, and inside out. This process is the same for healing skinned knees as it is for recovering from any condition you can name. If it's going to happen, you will become well from the inside.

*You may be wondering right now what's wrong with treating a problem from the outside in, with pills or other medication for example.   I would answer possibly nothing is wrong with that, in fact, it may be necessary to get you through the day or even to save a life in some instances. But this kind of treatment, based on "tire patch" mentality has **never** made anyone healthy and it never will.*

Think what a different world we'd have if the pharmaceutical giants weren't spending a billion dollars every month on massive ad campaigns. Yet, they spend those dollars so that you and I will believe that whenever we have an ache or pain, the right, moral, and ethical thing to do is run for the pill bottle. The school teacher has her pills, the cop on the beat has his pills, mom and dad have their medications, the priest, minister, and rabbi are all popping pills, and why not, with the clever and misleading ads they are running. "Plop-plop-fizz-fizz-oh-what-a-relief-it-is." The message is clear, go ahead stuff yourself, abuse your body, just take these pills, never mind the consequences. None of these treatments strengthen your Life-force.

Even more frightening are the prescriptions for antibiotics that poison your body.   Now we find out that they are, 1) virtually useless in fighting most infections, and 2) by taking them we (you) are advancing the mutations of these little microscopic beasts to the point that we are creating super breeds of bacteria! I recently read about a strain of bacteria that have evolved into a flesh-consuming breed. This has largely occurred thanks to antibiotics that have always killed most, **but not all** of the bacteria. The few that always remain after a dosage of antibiotics become more resilient and adaptable to modern medicine's futile efforts. The antibiotic treatments speed the process of natural selection up to light speed. Surviving bugs seem to love penicillin and tetracycline and all the other "super drugs" we throw at them.

"Tell a lie enough times and the lie becomes the truth." How did Adolph Hitler know that the drug companies would profit from his ideas and philosophies? No bigger lies have been perpetrated on the American public than the ideas formed by the self -serving pharmaceutical corporate world, as they shove down our throats (in the form of entertaining/ informative commercials and even news clips) the necessity for their poisons. Organized medicine has been "brain washing" us so well, and for so long (mostly through television) that their lies have become the "truth." In our society we have been subconsciously taught that it is ethically, morally, and physiologically correct to ingest chemical concoctions. We even serve these poisons to our children in the noble pursuit of numbing nerve endings or killing off a few select bacteria, all in the name of "health." Barely a nickel is spent in an attempt for you to discover ways to amplify your inborn health potential. If you think I sound a little strong on this subject... you're beginning to grasp my concern. Any time you end up in the hospital, your welfare is in jeopardy. Perhaps not necessarily from the treatment a doctor may administer, but from secondary infections that you may occasionally see written up in the newspapers and magazines. A 1995 Article from the *Quad-City Times*, points out what you seldom hear in today's media: that 180,000 people are killed every year in United States hospitals from improper medications and treatments (including surgery). It pointed out that medical error is a major killer in America, claiming more victims every year than violent crime and car accidents combined! To give you an idea of what that means, the airlines would have to *crash three jumbo jets every other day, throughout the entire year, to kill 180,000 people*! Let's keep you out of the hospital -- IT'S NOT SAFE IN THERE! Let's get well and stay healthy! We're getting close to the Big Idea.

SEE IF THESE CONCEPTS MAKE SENSE TO YOU:

Your body is like a self-cleaning oven. Given a chance, it will do all it can to clean up your internal mess.

This living human body has an innate, inborn desire to be well.

With the Life-force, your body has the potential to produce all the hormones and chemicals known, and unknown, at the right time, in the right amount. Your body then distributes these substances to the right places, without side effects, as long as we haven't interfered with the process.

This body was created by the most magnificent wisdom in the universe (if you don't believe that, we evolved over millions of years). Regardless of your orientation, I think you will agree that the human body is a miracle.

Lastly, the central nervous system (brain and spinal cord) is the master control system chosen to run and regulate all systems and organs of this wonderful gift, our body -- our life.

By the way, when I mention that the brain runs and regulates all the systems and all the organs, I'm certainly not suggesting that the brain you think with is responsible for the production and distribution of white corpuscles, testosterone, estrogen, respiration, metabolism, the digestion of food, etc. I'm told that just one single liver cell (under the influence and direction of your Life-force), needs to perform over one thousand different tasks per second in order to keep things going. Yet, you have billions of liver cells all working in symphony with the others to keep you alive. Would you want to trust your "conscious" brain with all of the functions for the heart, kidneys, pancreas, bowels, and the lungs? What would happen if you forgot to tell your heart to keep pumping while you slept? Why... you'd wake up the next morning.......dead! Personally, I'm glad it's not my conscious brain that is responsible for all this. Things would really be a mess inside my body otherwise. Just to prove the point, my wife gives me a list (to assist my conscience brain) of things to do.... I end up forgetting where I put the list! What a mind! I live by the saying "a short pencil is better than a long memory," not always in my case.

The cerebral hemispheres (the part that most people recognize as *the* brain) is the thinking, calculating, and "awake brain," but it is also really the "baby brain," even though one may have three college degrees and an I.Q. of 195. This brain was an open book of blank pages at birth- it knew nothing. In my case it has, however, accumulated a smattering of knowledge over a few decades, allowing me to put my thoughts on paper. Your brain allows you to comprehend and interpret, which is really a pretty neat process.

But the brain that I'm referring to contains the wisdom of the ages. It is the giant within. It knew at birth as much as it knows now. It is this brain that controls the beating of your heart, the digestion of food, and the production of hormones and chemicals. This unsung hero literally keeps you going. When you ingest or inhale an environmental toxin or foreign body such as viri or bacterium, this part of your brain utilizing your Life-force allows you to adapt. It is this portion of your brain that mounts the counter attack on a microscopic level. When your systems are working properly, the intruders are neutralized without your conscious mind ever having a clue. Besides, you're too busy getting the kids to school and dealing with the events of the day to know all, or even a portion , of what's really going on inside.

When a baby is born, (when <u>you</u> were born) this brain through the expression of the Life-force caused you to suckle when the nipple was near your mouth. You didn't have to take a class to learn how- fortunately, you just knew. This power is with you today as it recreates life on a daily basis. Liver and heart cells die off every 120 days (as they're prone to do), and they hopefully are replaced by new vibrant cells to help you continue your journey in life.

Many people, including some in the scientific world, take a mechanistic view to the whole thing by labeling these skills you've been given as "instinct" and "the workings of the subconscious brain." What a joke! Just because science can't tap into it, we have to label it as being beneath us, less than conscious. There is nothing subconscious about this healing mind. It is more correctly stated that this healing brain is <u>supra</u>-conscious. It's estimated that this "supra-conscious" brain, when functioning properly, is responsible for

5 to 6 Trillion functions every second! The tasks performed by it are simply incomprehensible by you and me. This is a major portion of the "Big Idea."

The greatest scientists, past, present, and future, will never fully understand the mysteries of the innate Life-force. The part of the brain that I'm referring to is called the brain stem. The brain stem has to do with all of these functions. If you happen to be suffering from chronic headache, you may also have a low level of vitality. You may not actually notice it yet, but your symptoms may be an indication that your immune system is not functioning at its best. There are numerous other conditions associated with the brain stem, and it is wise that you be aware of the implications of this very important region.

Some parts of the scientific community are taking on less of a mechanistic view, and are beginning to lean toward a more vitalistic approach to their investigations. These are the same scientists you might read about in *NewsWeek*, or *U.S.A. TODAY*. They explain that when farmers use a certain pesticide, in addition to the pesticide being ingested by you, the consumer, it not only kills the aphids and lady bugs, but the frogs and swallows that thrived on these bugs. And, because the frogs and swallows are absent, we have a bumper crop of flies and mosquitoes. These vitalistic scientists know (as you do) that when you just treat the symptoms, you invariably cause a whole set of new effects, upsetting the balance of nature. That observation is true whether you're looking at the external world, such as treating a farm with pesticides, or treating the internal environment of your body with chemicals.

This Innate Intelligence, resident in our Life-force not only keeps us alive (no wonder the drug companies haven't told us about it), it is systematic and uncluttered. It is your "Life-force" that keeps you breathing while you sleep. You are able to digest your food, manufacture estrogen, testosterone, and interferon. In fact, some of you can even grow babies without reading a book or even consciously thinking about it! This Innate Intelligence must be close to God.

LET'S GO BACK TO THE BEGINNING ... BEFORE YOU WERE YOU!

When we look at life unfold, we really are looking at-and living, a miracle. Two dabs of jelly are united (a sperm and an egg), and although science can't explain it, this is the beginning of a perfect human being-you! This fertilized dab of jelly is called a zygote. The zygote has all of the genetic blueprints necessary to build a perfect human being in about 280 days. The zygote splits and what was one cell, now has become two identical cells. Those two identical cells split, and now there are four. Four cells become eight, eight become sixteen, sixteen become thirty-two, thirty-two become sixty-four, one hundred twenty eight, two hundred fifty six, and on and on. All of them are perfect copies of the original single cell. This wildly expanding group of cells continue the mirror image duplication, until a particular time a few weeks later. Now certain cells begin to change. This is the beginning of a process called "differentiation and specialization."

I have to stop for a moment and point something out. Up to now, all of the cells of the embryo are genetically identical.

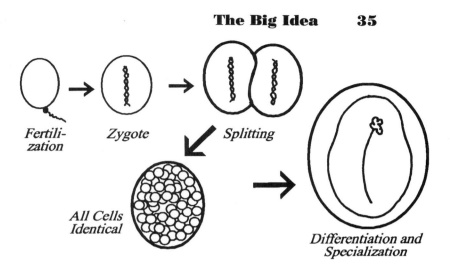

Fertili-
zation   Zygote   Splitting

All Cells
Identical

Differentiation and
Specialization

But, through the unexplainable process of "differentiation and specialization," certain cells become different. The first cells that change logically become the precursors to the system that runs the whole show. A little bud develops at one end of the embryo, then a stem trails away from the bud (inset). This is the beginning of your brain and spinal cord.

As growth continues, some cells that are changing become liver cells, and they grow where the liver will be. Other cells specialize into kidney, lung or heart cells, and each do their specialized duties. Wouldn't it be terrible if we were just a big blob of one type of cell? No headaches perhaps, but life would really be boring, we'd be like a multi-cellular amoeba. We'd probably just be taking up space, totally incapable of thinking or having any initiative. We would consume all masses smaller than us, and we'd be consumed by those larger than us! Actually, that sounds a little like some "couch potatoes" I personally know.

Back to "differentiation and specialization." I find it fascinating that the first cells that change in the embryo develop into the one organ that must regulate the growth and development of all other cells and organs. This new type of cell forms the beginning of the most delicate, yet the most powerful system we have. It's the one system that doesn't replace itself (at least not very easily). It's the one organ that runs roughshod over the developing organs and systems of this tiny embryo, and, fortunately, doesn't abandon us once we leave the womb.

Can you guess?

I hope you're not guessing now. You know that this most powerful system is the brain and nerve system. It's rather puzzling how there is a Heart Foundation, an American Cancer Society, and, of course, "Jerry's Kids" for the Muscular Dystrophy Foundation. It's sad that society has no huge, visible program for the Innate Intelligence Foundation. After all, every other disease that you can name is directly connected to how well your body is connected to, and expressing, its inherent organizational abilities. There are many causes of specific disease and maladies, but the one major cause of disharmony in the body may go undetected for decades while setting the stage for any and every disease or malady you could name. It's true, there really should be a foundation for the full expression of one's Innate Intelligence. A "Life-force" foundation if you will. This would be the ultimate form of health care, to ensure that 5 to 6 trillion life-protecting functions per second, on a cellular basis, are working in symphony to protect you in a way that is light-years ahead of anything that "modern" disease treatment can offer.

NOW YOU'RE READY !

The Big Idea is that you've got it *all* within you, although someone with chronic headaches may not believe that just yet. And, the Big Idea doesn't necessarily deal with treatments and cures- it's more a state of mind that dispells fear, as my friend Dr. Fred Barge calls it in his book, *Life Without Fear.*

The Big Idea includes the realization that this living body is better able to respond if the nerve system is wide open and fully connected. The Big Idea is understanding that you're better off *with* your tonsils, appendix, and uterus (although it sometimes has been necessary to remove them to save life) than without them. If these organs *have* been removed, then the Big Idea becomes even more important (if that's possible). Now, with missing pieces of anatomy, one should do more of the "right" things to ensure that the parts you do have are working at their level best. **Remember**, health is defined as a condition of **Wholeness** in which all of the parts are **Functioning** at optimum capacity. So it is vital to keep as many of our parts as we can, and keep them working well from above, down, and inside out (ADIO).

Some of the people that I've consulted who are suffering from chronic headache (and other serious conditions) behave in a manner totally consistent with a form of denial.

Because they're under a doctor's care or on "medication," they behave as if they're excused from reality. You've heard these people say, "Oh, my doctor has me on (whatever medication)," and they act as if everything else going on in the body is on hold. There can be a false sense of security when one denies that there may be consequences in continuous medications. They disengage (mentally) from the Big Idea. They have forgotten that health is an inside job, and over a time of living in the medical drug culture one moves further from the possibility of embracing the laws of life. For these people "a natural life style" is great material to *talk* about, but they need someone or something to show them their folly, and re-introduce them to the Big Idea. They'll actually get a glimpse of their lie when they are asked certain questions. Momentarily they'll realize the rules of life: Cause and effect are still fully engaged.   Ask one of your distant relatives...

HOW'S YOUR HEALTH? (they answer)
     "Fine."
NO, REALLY, HOW'S YOUR HEALTH?
          "Oh, you mean my health?"
YES, YOUR HEALTH, HOW IS IT?
                    "Well, I have bleeding ulcers but
                    I'm on medication for that. Other
                    than my bleeding ulcers I'm in
                    perfect health."

WOW, do you know someone like that?

Let's now clearly define our "Big Idea" ... it is the concept that you were born with all the health potential you'll ever have. If we pretty much live a non-destructive lifestyle, we will likely heal better and last longer. There is a self-righting mechanism at work within your body that's under the direction of your inborn Life-force (which flows through the nervous system). The people who are under medical treatment are the people who most desperately need to study and embrace the six foundational keys for health amplification. Unfortunately, they are usually the least likely to take heed unless, *or until*, something goes sour in their medical treatment.

You now more fully understand... you've got all you need inside to be healthy, so let's try to use the safest, most delicate approach to untangle the mess you may be in. And, in addition to just treating an obvious headache condition, let's also strive to amplify the good within, and amplify the Life-force.

To better understand the absolute validity of all this, I want to arm you with the artillery you'll need to protect yourself from your friends, family, and yes, even your doctors. You will leave them in awe, totally defenseless, quivering in fear of your new found wisdom and vision. To prepare you for the 6 foundational keys to health amplification, we should first give you a short course on ......

• Chapter Five •

INDUCTIVE AND DEDUCTIVE REASONING

"Everyone is ignorant, only on different subjects."
--Will Rogers

It's 9:30 A.M. on Sunday morning, in fact, it's Mother's Day and we're just relaxing around the house. The phone rings. My wife, Pauli, answers it. "Hi," she says, "oh, happy Mother's Day to you, too!" I'm thinking it's either her sister or one of our moms. They chat for awhile and, then, my ears perk up. Pauli repeats what she has just heard on the phone for my entertainment. I know that because she's looking right at me with the phone to her ear, as she repeats, "You're taking something now, to undo what the antibiotics did <u>to</u> you?" That's all I had to hear. I knew it was one of the three ladies, and I knew I would hear more.

I later found out that her mom had developed an ear infection. She had been prescribed, and swallowed, a regime of pills to do battle with the infection. However, as an added bonus of consuming the antibiotics, her mom was left with a massive, itching and oozing rash on her right leg. This rash now required its own medical treatment with a variation of a cortisone drug.

The sequence was one medical treatment leading to a new problem, which required yet another form of damaging treatment. This is not a new phenomenon! We've acknowleged that all drugs and medications have side effects. Some of these side effects (from headaches to liver and kidney damage) are more pronounced than others, often requiring a more dangerous intervention the second or third time around.

Today, surgery in hospitals can lead to infections (often staph infections) so resistant to antibiotics that the secondary problem is often worse than the original condition. Secondary complications can occasionally be fatal. You may know of someone (perhaps close to you) who died as a result of a drug "reaction." There is a name for this phenomenon... any time you or a family member becomes ill as a result of medical treatment, the newly <u>induced</u> condition is said to be an *IATROGENIC* disease.

Iatrogenic diseases are running out of control in the "developed" nations of the world. The World Health Organization reported a few years ago that approximately 80 percent of all diseases today result from the treatment of some other disease condition. For example, if you or a family member had a kidney condition (you could pick headache) and you were put on a treatment program of medication (chemicals), the medication may help the kidneys, or whatever organ it was designed for. However, while this chemical is working on the target organ, it is also flowing through your blood stream, poisoning previously innocent healthy organs. And, while this chemical may be medicinal to your kidneys or your head pain, it may be an extreme poison to your liver or heart, and other parts of the body. The result ... some level of reaction that has the potential to produce an *Iatrogenic disease,* if the reaction, over time, is strong enough. There is a chance that your headaches are are totally or partially iatrogenic in origin.

The prefix "iatro" means *physician*. "Genic," like genesis means the *beginning of*. So, by definition, iatrogenic literally means physician-induced disease. Perhaps with all the talk about health care reform, while attempting to save lives and money, someone should put a spotlight on this hidden epidemic. Iatrogenic disease is a concept you need to be aware of for your own safety.

Side note: The cover of the March 28, 1994 issue of Newsweek read, *ANTIBIOTICS the end of miracle drugs*. The article described how microbes are increasingly becoming resistant. And that antibiotics will be completely useless in a few years. The abuse of medications, not limited to antibiotics, is a massive cause of iatrogenic disease in our culture. The best defense is a good offense, meaning: *"Keep your own immune system at peak performance,"* which is *exactly* what we're hoping to help you do.

How did our society get into such a mess? Today it is so common for "health care" to be the cause of so many problems that we don't even think it's unusual! The answer must lie in the way we have been taught to think. Let's take a look at **inductive** and **deductive** reasoning. An understanding of the two will help set you free when dealing with doctors, friends and even family while discussing your health.

First, let's examine **inductive** reasoning. Pure scientific projects require induction. Math is a pure science, it deals with inanimate objects ... there is no real need for adaptability or variables (you are not dealing with living organisms). Two plus two always equals four. And as a result of that, one can induce that doubling the numbers will give a proportionate result: 4+4=8. It always has and it always will. These formulas are truths, they are immutable and unwavering.

Inductive reasoning is that process in which one can take a small sampling, i.e. 2+2=4, and induce that since it is true, then, it must also be true on a larger scale: 200+200=400. In math this seems to hold up. Chemistry is another pure science where inductive thinking works well. Chemical "A" mixed with chemical "B" always yields a new chemical "C," under like circumstances. This always seems to be true whether on a minute or grand scale.

Numbers are not alive; there is no need to consider individuality or unique characteristics. Likewise, chemicals behave exactly the same way all the time. Therefore, **inductive** reasoning is perfect for a pure science, but is seriously flawed when considering a person's health. You're now dealing with a variable, a *living* being. Can it be possible that you still have headaches because the appropriate treatment for you doesn't fit into some national average? Could you possibly need a unique or specialized approach to your individual problem? Unfortunately, someone long ago decided that the scientific method was the only valid way of dealing with people's health. **But, people are not numbers, each of us are very unique, and we respond differently in similar situations.** We are equally as different on the inside as we are on the outside!

From a health and healing standpoint, here is where inductive thinking has gotten us. A study was performed on a few hundred people several decades ago. This study revealed that the *average* body temperature in the group was 98.6 degrees Fahrenheit. That was the *average*, not the best or the normal. However, over the years, 98.6 degrees has become the expected norm. It is often implied that if you are above or below that temperature you must be sick! This average temperature has little to do with reality. Your "normal" may run a few degrees high or low because, after all, you are an individual with unique factors. Inductive thinking doesn't allow much for these inherent variables.

What if you mistakenly eat some food that is spoiled. If your body is healthy and responding accordingly, I should think your temperature might well rise to burn up invading microbes. Would you be comfortable as your body temperature rises? Probably not. Would you be sick? One might "think" so, as you may feel pretty bad with sweating, perhaps vomiting ... but I contend you are not sick. Rather, your body is responding in an efficient manner to an ingested toxin. Your Life-force knows that those bugs can't survive the heat. You may certainly feel like you are sick, but your body is doing the best it can if you'll just give it a chance. Once again, remember that health has to do with function, and these body parts are functioning at high capacity to clean themselves out. Amazing!

Bringing down the temperature artificially, or drinking some pink potion to coat an "upset" stomach, can prolong the distress. In other words, your body has some intelligence. Conventional inductive beliefs, however, would define your rising temperature as a malfunction. Science would attempt to bring down the fever, prolonging a favorable environment for the microbes, allowing them to spread the infection throughout your body.

Inductive reasoning also results in the belief that we should all have a blood pressure reading of 120 over 80. This is so absurd, I hardly know where to begin. First, I'll share a couple of exceptions to this. If you are getting a blood pressure reading and you have a full bladder, your reading could be off by 15 points or more. You may be nervous about being in the doctor's office, thus, raising your blood pressure. If your doctor is hard of hearing his incorrect reading could add another 10 points. And, just because someone said 120 over 80 is the average, it certainly doesn't make it normal or healthy for you. Your normal, this year may be 110 over 70 and next year it could be 130 over 90.

One more example of inductive thinking. Have you ever looked at the nutritional information supplied by the government on a cereal box? On the side it will read Minimum Daily Requirements of certain vitamins, minerals, protein, and other nutrients. Who are these people? And, how do they know what I need? Do you believe, for a moment, that you and I have the same minimum nutritional needs? No way! Could Bobby Shoemaker, the great Kentucky Derby jockey weighing in around 100 pounds, have the same needs as Shaquille O'Neill, the NBA's premiere 300-pound, 7 foot-*plus* center? Of course not! In fact, you have different nutritional needs today than you did yesterday. My body, like yours, is always changing and adapting moment to moment, day to day. Your body is either adapting and growing stronger, or weakening and breaking down. The nutritional components needed don't necessarily reflect the inductive concept of lumping us together into averages.

The bottom line... there are just too many variables and individualities to study only a small group and *induce* conclusions about the remaining population. You and I are individuals and we usually don't fit into national averages.

Now, here's the other side of the coin. **Deductive** reasoning is far from perfect but it seems to have a broader application for dealing with an individual's health.

Deductive thought processes first require a major premise. Christianity provides an interesting example. It has a major premise, or a major big idea. This being that God is Omnipotent, and wants the best for his children. That's a pretty broad statement but it's where deduction starts -- a large assumption that we can move from. It leads you to deduce specific information or considerations about an individual or a situation. Also, God's existence is a belief or an assumption. I can't prove it to you, so there must be some agreement in this process (by the way, I also can't prove that 2+2=4, so there must also be agreement with inductive reasoning as well).

Taking the broad, agreed-upon belief that God loves all of mankind, an individual can apply that grand belief to his or her life. One can then deduce ways to fashion his or her daily life and activities around this major premise.

If, however, a major premise is incorrect, the resulting deductions will be equally false. Our ancestors, for example, believed that the earth was flat and that the earth sat in the center of the solar system. They believed that the sun and stars rotated around us. As a result of that flawed major premise, the maps and navigation of the day were quite inaccurate.

> ## PREMISE:
> I have *some* health.
> ## DEDUCTION:
> *If I amplify the health I have, I can feel BETTER, have more fun, and enjoy life MORE!*

So, deductive reasoning goes from the general (big picture) down to the specific individual case. Inductive reasoning flows the opposite direction, from the specific small sample (like the 500 people in the blood pressure study), up to a conclusion on how you and I, and the rest of the world, should fit into the rank and file. Inductive reasoning tells us we should behave ourselves and not be different. Sounds sort of like a basis for socialized health care, doesn't it?

Now that we have an understanding of inductive and deductive thinking, we can get down to business, knowing that for the most part we will be using a deductive process. The major premise (Big Idea) for this work is really quite simple, and I think you'll find it quite reasonable. There is within each of us an intelligence that is working at all times for our survival. This Intelligence or Life-force exists in all our tissues and cells, and when the Life-force is fully expressing itself our body is more fully alive and better able to adapt to the environment. When the Life-force is not intact, malfunction, disease and eventual death of all or part, of the organism can occur.

The Life-force is there when your child scrapes his or her knee, and without "treatment" the wisdom within instantly sends a repair team to the sight of injury. The Life-force within you directs the digestion of the midnight snack you ate. Perhaps you had a peanut butter sandwich.... instead of rotting in your gut, the Life-force within takes this gooey mess and turns it into skin, brain and liver cells or what ever tissues you might be needing. What a wonderful body! When the Life-force is present, your body is constantly performing miracles, which are far too reaching for any of us to fully understand. This is deductive thinking. I believe there is a Life-force within (major premise), and I have evidence to support my belief. Happily, this deductive line of thought can provide you a lot of personal power when dealing with health issues in your life.

Even when a person is extremely ill, for instance with cancer, one might notice that there is an apparent lack of adaptability and Life-force in the person's body, leaving them looking pale and drawn. Why? Perhaps the Life-force is drawing their body's resources into the site of the disease. The reserves of the body are being spent in an obvious effort to do battle, to avoid being overtaken. Now you know why that person may look gaunt. Just consider the recuperative powers of the body being summoned inside for repair rather than on outward appearance.

In summary, there is an internal wisdom at work in every living body, a Life-force that is working to insure survival and wellness. That will be our basic premise, or bottom-line belief, for the deductive processes we are about to explore. It is through the meeting of your reasoning process, our gentle technology and your Life-force that we are able to allow you to begin the healing process. I know this is different than how you've looked at yourself and your health in the past. But I am hopeful that you are reading this to gain a new, different, and better result in your life experience. The words of Albert Einstein remind us that, "To continue to do the same things over and over again, and to expect a new result, now that's insanity." So, if some of what you read in this book seems a little weird, rather than ignore or condemn it, let's celebrate your discovery of new data and technology designed to amplify the wealth of reserves within.

To maximize the expression of this Life-force is certainly in your best interest. This leads us to **Foundational Key #1**. To begin to amplify your health, you must provide your cells with plenty of...

• Chapter Six •

AIR
Foundational Key #1

"Breathing ... the first step to a clean bloodstream."
-- Dr. Jeff Finnigan

In order to heal and regain your health, you'll need a surplus of energy to assist in the healing process. Perhaps more correctly stated, you'll need to *generate* more energy than you have in the past. It is, in fact, entirely possible that you are in your current situation (at least in part) due to a lack of energy. And now we need to increase your body's energy output.

So where does energy come from? It does not come from candy bars or greasy hamburgers! In fact, it actually doesn't come from nutritious foods either. Often times, when I am invited to give a talk on alternative health measures, my prospective audience assumes that I am going to speak on nutrition. I eventually do, but to establish a hierarchy of importance I ask the audience this question. "How long can you live without consuming food?" The answer is you can go without food for weeks. Then I ask, "how long can you go without consuming oxygen?" At this point, the group understands that it is correct to discuss the role of proper oxygenation of the body before we venture into further areas.

Most people don't realize that within a given period of time, their body consumes more air than food and water combined! So, just like food and water you are a "consumer" of air, and you should be somewhat picky about its quality. Some sources of air are more polluted than others; try not to live your life downwind from a pulp mill or right next to a freeway. You may choose to avoid certain foods that have chemical preservatives or chemical taste enhancers such as MSG, because you have experienced undesirable reactions to these substances. Perhaps you completely avoid them because you realize, in the long run, your life will be more enhanced without these concoctions. A similar consideration should be given to your air consumption.

You also may have a water filtration system in your home. On May 12th, 1993, *USA Today* announced on the front page, that according to the EPA, 819 U.S. cities have water systems containing unhealthy levels of lead! The list of cities continues to grow. This type of situation unwittingly effects millions upon millions of us and can thwart our efforts for health and recovery. By the way, lead is only one of many pathogenic agents that can flow through our tap water. It is important that the nutrients we consume, along with the water and air, are as pure as possible.

But breathing air is so obvious, it's involuntary, so why would I even bring it into the equation? Because so many of us breathe in a way that disempowers rather than oxygenates our bodies. Even though you breathe without a thought, chances are you have become accustomed to breathing in a way that does not provide all the power that is available to you. Oh, by the way, to answer my earlier question about where energy comes from...

BREATHING PROVIDES POWER AND ENERGY, AND ALSO ENHANCES MENTAL CLARITY.

Even your automobile "knows" that it produces greater energy with more air. Did you know that when you're cruising down the highway and you put your foot on the accelerator, you're not just giving the engine more gas, but also adding air to the combustion process? Without air, there is no life in the performance of your car. Without air, there is no life in the performance of your body!

In northern parts of the country, where wood stoves are popular, you'll notice that once the fire is going, a baffle is used to control how hot or cool your fire will burn. The baffle controls only the flow of air to the fire. The consumption of oxygen makes all the difference as to how the fire burns both in the stove ... and in your body. The performance of your body on a cellular level is influenced by your oxygen intake and has much to do with your ability to heal and stay well.

Here are a couple of interesting fast facts for you. I'm informed that one in three Americans will contract cancer in his or her lifetime. I've seen statistics that only one in seven athletes will contract cancer in their lifetime. What a huge statistical difference! That's a gigantic discrepancy! So what is the difference between you and me, and athletes? Massive volumes of oxygen! They run and jump and run some more. They swim, lift weights and they run some more. My point is, after running the 100-yard dash and swimming for 25 minutes continuously, the body demands huge volumes of oxygen.

Your cells need to be bathed in oxygen to be healthy and vibrant.

I could, at this point, digress and try to explain how the CO_2 and O_2 are exchanged in the alveoli of the lungs and how the hemoglobin carries these gases throughout the blood stream, but there are plenty of texts for that purpose. Instead, let's review the work Otto Warburg, Nobel Prize winner and director of the Planck Institute for Cell Physiology, and later, what Dr. H. Goldblatt collaborated in the *Journal of Experimental Medicine.* It described how simply by lowering the oxygen content available to cells from rats, cellular functions were altered to the point of slowing down the metabolism. This caused some cells to die while causing other cells, because of the alteration in metabolism, to mutate and even become malignant. Thus, breathing techniques are very important. And, it is certainly possible that the way a person breathes could contribute to headache.

Other lifestyle choices that people unwittingly make hinder the oxygen availability to cells. Can you guess what they might be? Obviously, smoking tobacco pollutes the internal environment. There are around 50 million smokers in the United States who are, to some level, addicted. Millions of deaths each year are directly related to smoking. Smoking interferes with the hemoglobin's ability to properly bind to oxygen and carry it to the cells. There are vast amounts of documentation about the detrimental effects of smoking, so I will not belabor this point. And, I don't want to be misunderstood.

I'm <u>not</u> saying that in order for you to get well, or for you to adopt these methods, you have to give up this habit. There are hundreds of thousands of people who live long and productive lives while smoking a pack or two per day. But, I will offer reasoning in the next chapter as to why they are able to "get away with it."   You must also know that your chances vastly improve when you clean up your lungs.

What are some other less obvious inhibitors to our oxygen absorption ... how about fatty foods and excess salt?

Not only can fatty foods make you fat, they also thicken the blood stream. Fatty foods make the red blood cells sticky ... resulting in a sluggish transport of oxygen through the system. Imagine your arteries as a crystal clear mountain stream flowing freely through its channels. This vision should represent the normal, healthy flow of your oxygen-carrying capacity (remember, the duty of your red blood cells is to carry oxygen to the distant recesses of your body) by your arterial supply. Then, unfortunately, someone has a toxic waste spill somewhere up stream!   This mess (probably caused by a cheeseburger, some fries and a shake) turns the once free-flowing stream into an oozing, slow, sloppy mess that no longer efficiently does what it is designed to do.

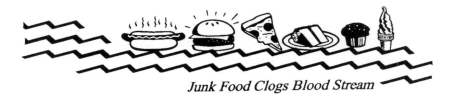

Junk Food Clogs Blood Stream

In addition to the slowing and sticking of the red blood cells, this fatty mess also sticks to the inside walls of the arteries to form the beginnings of plaque. This plaquing of the inner walls, as you can visualize, results in a tighter hole for the blood to flow through. Now, because the blood vessels have a smaller internal diameter, the heart must use more pressure to pump the blood, thus, <u>creating</u> *high blood pressure*! Now the heart is working harder to accomplish the same task it has always done with less effort, and you have the makings of an honest-to-goodness diagnosable condition called Cardio-vascular Disease. This is a simplification of the process, but can you see the interconnectedness of the internal living environment? *(We're not just treating you for headache pain.)*

By affecting one area of the body, you automatically influence all other organs and systems. In the above scenario, we only mentioned the bloodstream, the heart and the arteries. But you soon realize that this type of condition is much more far reaching in its consequences. The liver, kidneys, pancreas and everything inside of you will have to alter their <u>functions</u> (there's that word again) in order to adapt and compensate for the obvious hindrance to the oxygen transport system.

By the way, this adaptation is coordinated by the Life-force that is inherent in your living nerve system. "Houston Control" has no better back-up system than what you and I have been given as a gift. We really should say "thank you" for these gifts on a regular basis. We probably should take better care of this wonderful equipment, too.

Self -Help Activities: There are a few good ways to increase the oxygen levels in your body. One of the easiest ways, which I frequently use for myself, is to take in a huge breath of air, as much as one can comfortably inhale. Hold it for 30 or 60 seconds, feeling the increased pressure in your lungs and tension against the inside of your rib cage. Release the air slowly through pinched lips, then quickly take a deep cleansing breath and then briskly blow it out. This will assist in creating an oxygen rich environment where oxygen is defusing and being filtered to your blood stream. Be sure to be sitting down when experimenting with this breathing technique, for it is possible to become dizzy if you hold your air too long in the beginning. Don't try to set any records, at least for now. All we want to do is start waking up your cells and bringing them back to life. If you have a cardiovascular or respiratory condition, you should consult your physician on this breathing technique before you begin. This breathing technique frequently helps many headache sufferers. Even if you don't notice a measurable improvement quickly, please know that everyone responds at their own rate. Even if breathing doesn't reduce your pain, your overall health can only benefit from the improved oxygenation!

This deep diaphragmatic breathing technique not only helps create the oxygen availability that your body is looking for, but will also pump your lymph system. The lymph system is the sewage and garbage transport system of the body. Unfortunately, it has no automatic pumping mechanism like the heart. If the lymph becomes stagnated, you have cellular waste (garbage) accumulating in your bodily humors (liquids). This garbage transport system requires muscular activity, and as I mentioned, deep diaphragmatic breathing will stimulate the cleansing effect. When a person is ill for an extended period of time, consider the jeopardizing effect of inactivity. The individual feels bad to begin with, so there is a tendency to lay low, to sit or even remain in bed. Because he or she is inactive and likely to be breathing very shallowly, in addition to all the other concerns, we now have a stagnating lymph system, contributes to a more toxic internal environment. With a lack of empowered breathing techniques a process of auto-intoxication ensues, further hampering recovery. At the very least, proper oxygenation of our tissues has to take a position of paramount importance for the healthy to stay well, and for the ill to better recover. Air is still free, there is no charge! You are entitled to as much as you can "stomach." So go ahead on this one ... be a pig! The more good clean air you consume, the better off you'll be.

CONCLUSION: The quality and quantity of air that you consume has a direct impact on the state of the organism (you). *Air* is Foundational Key #1 to Reigniting your Life-force.

ACTION STEP: Breath in a way that is *empowering*, not just *sustaining*.

Of course you remember George Burns, the great cigar-smoking comedian who lived 100 glorious years. How is it that some people go through life, breaking all the rules, with poor eating, drinking and smoking habits, yet seem to be healthy? They never miss any work, and they live a long productive life. How is it that they can do all the fun stuff and "get away" with it? That just doesn't seem fair!

To answer that question we'll take a little side trip before we discuss **Foundational Key #2**. Let's explore ......

• Chapter Seven •

THE LINCH PIN THEORY OF
HEALTH AND DISEASE

*"The man who removes a mountain begins by
carrying away small stones."*
--Chinese Proverb

My clinical observations and investigations have led me to
the conclusion that on a physical plane, there are six **Foundational Keys to Health Amplification**.

It seems nearly every day you can read in the newspaper or
hear through the "grapevine," that a university medical research team has come up with a new cure for one disease or
another. Aunt Tilly has a cure for the common cold or the
common hangover. The world is full of these remedies. For
every condition you can name, from cancer to ingrown toe
nails, someone has "the Answer" for us.

I don't mean to make light of these cures, whether home-
brewed or from the most sophisticated labs on the planet,
because many of them do work for certain people. But don't
you get just a little bit suspicious when they keep coming up
with these "cures," yet people still get sick with the same diseases? In the 1970's President Richard Nixon allocated hundreds of millions of tax dollars to cure and eradicate cancer.
Still we have a multitude of charitable organizations pander-
ing for our donations so that "this" won't happen to you and
yours. In reality, we are light years away from predictably

curing cancer. With all the research money and time spent, cancer is as frightening today as it was 30 years ago!

Now we have a new monster disease called AIDS. In full-blown cases, cancer often attacks at the end to finish off these poor souls. Can you guess where the billions of tax dollars are being directed in research today? That's right, the Center for Disease Control is trying to figure out a way to kill the HIV virus, as if it has been proven that the HIV virus *causes* the disease.

But you see, if the virus causes AIDS, then it should cause the disease all, *or at least most*, of the time. Yet, there are thousands of people who were intimate with someone who had the disease, but the first person is clear of any trace of infection, let alone the disease. Two people may have exchanged body fluids for years, and the second person not only didn't get the disease, but the alleged pathogen, (the HIV virus) could not be found in his or her body! Further, there have been numerous surgeons who, while working on AIDS patients, accidentally lacerated or punctured their own finger, thus ensuring a bilateral exchange of blood. One would shudder at the thought of having this happen. It truly would have to be a doctor's worst nightmare, waiting weeks, months or even years later for results that came from the slip of his or her own hand. But, happily, in the vast majority of such cases no infection sets in, and no HIV virus is found.

I don't want you to misinterpret my intent. This chapter is not about AIDS or cancer or any one particular disease. In reality, this belief system and theory holds true for all health conditions and resultant diseases. In addition to addressing the subject of eliminating headaches, this chapter is about learning to live a "life without fear."

The same sort of occurrences have happened for decades in tuberculosis wards and in hospitals dealing with "highly" contagious diseases. Nurses and doctors may wear a strip of cloth across their mouths and noses, but this offers virtually no protection to the passage of bacteria and viruses. The pores in a surgical mask are like a freeway to microscopic organisms. Doctors and nurses breathe exactly the same air as the infected patients. In fact, they'll stand squarely in front of a patient, ask the patient to stick out his or her tongue and cough right into their face 10 inches away! Do the nurses and doctors then contract the disease? Hardly ever! You can't convince me that these people (the doctors) believe in the "germ theory" of disease. If the germ theory were true we'd all be sick, all the time. If the doctors believed that germs cause disease then there's no way that they would work in that environment for any amount of money... would you?

Finally, society is realizing that health is a multifaceted commodity. What I mean is that there are six (or more) major components, and your health needs are not the same today as they were yesterday. And they'll be different tomorrow. We're all changing all the time. Science will never understand all that goes on inside us. I simply make this observation so we can stand together in awe of the wonders of life.

There are **Foundational Keys**, or **Linch Pins** (the first is **AIR**), that we all have in common, and we need to examine them in a deductive and even an inductive way. Be assured that these six keys are extremely beneficial to all, regardless of headache or our present state of health. The more one relies upon and embraces these six keys, a broader foundation is created for our physiological well-being, and, incidentally, will also improve any of our other current health concerns.

Have you ever had a friend convince you to try her "cure all" health improvement program (from exercise machines to cancer -curing tea), because she just couldn't stop talking about the wondrous results she obtained? But when you tried it, you only ended up wasting precious time and money.

I have a theory as to why that happened to you. Consider the **Six Foundational Keys to Health and Disease**. You see, your friend who got wondrous results had all the other five keys turned to the "on" position and working for her. She had done enough "right things" to prepare her body for a quantum leap. Perhaps she stopped smoking seven months earlier. Maybe she got a new dog that required daily walks. She may not have even realized that she had prepared herself and she was ready. She was on the launching pad. Unwittingly, she was able to have an "over night" success with one event or one product. She may never realize that there had been a sequence of events that assisted her in having such noticeable results.

You, on the other hand, may need to turn three or four Foundational Keys to the "on" position before you can enjoy the same thunderous response of health amplification.

You are about to learn the Foundational Keys to amplifying your health for a lifetime. ***Warning*** ...you may start turning these keys to the "on" position and not initially recognize any noticeable improvements until you take the right actions long enough and engage more (or all) of the Keys to Health.

So what does this   mean?

It means I probably could rename this book *The Six Foundational Keys to Health*, because we are going way beyond just trying to provide you some relief from your headache pain. The beauty of this approach is that we work to get you on the launch pad by first acknowledging and then engaging these factors. This multiple key concept is the central and paramount theme for the Life-force principles. I can't really say that these ideas alone are revolutionary in principle. As you read and develop a full understanding of what's at hand, you likely won't fall off your chair with a new astounding cognition. But as you apply the six key approach to your overall health beliefs and lifestyle, your *results* can be astounding, revolutionary, even miraculous.

Foundational Keys

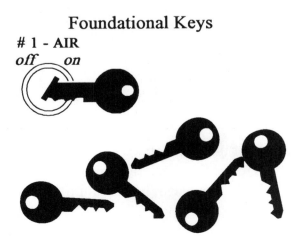

1 - AIR

off   *on*

These six factors will sound disarmingly simple at first. I've already told you about the first key-breathing. That certainly seems simple enough. You may tend to pass them all off as too easy, or you might think you've got it handled. Please, for your sake, take these valuable concepts to heart, become a student, and live these principles as they begin to make sense to you. The following dab of information, when *lived* and *adhered* to, could turn your world around.

The Six Foundational Keys simply imply that: For you to recover and stay well, you must engage all the critical Keys to **ALLOW** your body to function the way it was designed to.

"Health" is optimum function of all the parts of your body. Turning the keys to *"on"* is synonymous with removing interferences to the <u>function</u> of your body.

There is a principle in physiology that states that *all processes take time.* You can't "make" the body work right or recover immediately. Doctors can stimulate and speed up certain functions, and although that may be necessary to do on occasion, it's not uncommon to suffer serious side effects from powerful stimulants. In order for one's body to truly heal, an allotment of time must be entered into the equation.

Realizing the belief system that your body, if allowed to, strives to be well and remain in a state of dynamic balance, provides you with a world of opportunity to <u>assist,</u> rather than <u>force</u> a response, or a reaction, out of a malfunctioning portion of your body. Let me put it this way. Your body is a little bit like a compass: It is predictable and strives to stay on course. A compass, like your body, can get spun around and shaken up, but when left alone and allowed to respond it will "hunt" its way back to normal. If you take the right actions, your body will strive to balance things out on its own. You do the healing -- I'll remove barriers. This is teamwork. **Caution:** I am certainly not suggesting to someone in the final stages of serious disease that all we should do is step back and let the Life-force step in and clean up the mess. There are limitations to matter if damage and time are left to run unchecked. In other words, the disease process may have surpassed the ability of the organ (the matter) to rebound. This is seldom the case with chronic headaches, regardless of what you've been told, but these factors, can slow or complicate an otherwise speedy recovery.

Limitations of matter is an important concept. You may have an expensive engine in your automobile. If left sitting out in the elements, unprotected and unmaintained for a period of time, your engine would fill with corrosion and eventually be worthless. The body can only tolerate so much neglect. Hopefully, the neglect that your body has endured has now ceased and repair can now begin.

But health (not disease treatment) really is a simple and fun process. Health is a normal state, disease is abnormal. Health can be compared to daytime, where there is sunlight. Night is no different from daytime other than we have turned our backs on the sun. Night is an absence of light; add sunlight and you have day. Disease is an absence of health; add balance and Life-force, and you'll have improved health. Like the compass, given the chance our bodies will seek a balanced state.

The Earth itself is a lot like that, too. If we give her half a chance, with some passage of time trees will grow in an area of clear cutting and soon the wildlife will return. When we pollute the rivers and seas it appears that if we provide some clean-up efforts and allow time to pass, healing and a return to the natural thriving state will occur. The Life-force is self-perpetuating, and is here to serve your needs.

Below you will note a figure. It demonstrates the sequential effect of increased wellness as we engage the keys to the "on" position for our innate health potential. You have begun breathing in a way that is empowering, so you have meta-phorically turned the first key, putting you solidly on

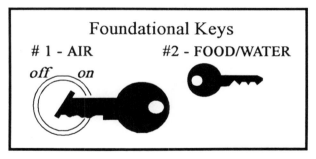

"first base." Now that you are here, you can't help but notice that staring you right in the face is Foundational Key #2. It's irresistible! You can't help yourself! Knowing that there is no other way to the next level in your quest for greater health without turning the next key, you firmly grab it and briskly engage it to the "on" position.

Isn't it refreshing that this theory is not about one miracle "cure-all" ? But, rather, a realistic approach about personal integrity and being responsible for oneself. We can turn these six keys and, with the momentum of our efforts and slightly altered lifestyles, be pulled up to higher, more efficient, internal biological functions.

As you begin to realize just exactly what key number two involves, you'll notice that it is the logical sequel to step one. "This is going to be so easy," you say to yourself. But remember what I said earlier, this will make all the sense in the world, and won't really seem revolutionary in <u>principle</u>. It will, however, be revolutionary in <u>practice</u>.

My wife and I always try to teach our children that no matter what the situation is, they always have options. So do you. Sometimes we get caught up in habits, rather than consider- ing our options. Let's see how we can use this next topic for healing, not just for entertainment and fulfillment. I'm talk- ing about one of my favorite distractions.
 I'll bet you like it, too. I'm referring to ...

• Chapter Eight •

FOOD AND WATER
Foundational Key #2

First, let's talk about water. I'd rather talk about food, but we'll save that for dessert. Next to air, water is number two in the hierarchy of important factors to sustain life. We can live without food for one or two months, but without water we'll only last a few days. For some patients their headache problems are triggered by a state of chronic dehydration, and several health problems are linked to low water intake.

How much of the planet do you suppose is covered by water? I am told about 70 to 80 percent. Think about the earth being composed mostly of water. It is easy to visualize the world as if you were looking from the moon. The vast blue oceans virtually blanket our earth. But water, even in middle America, is far away from the oceans... just look outside your window. You'll probably see some trees, hopefully some flowers and a variety of ground cover. What are all these plants composed of? Mostly water, about 70 to 90 percent, even though you don't see it.

How much of your body do you think is made up of water?

Again, I've seen numbers from 75 to 95 percent. Remarkable correlation, isn't it?

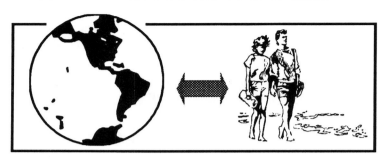

THE SURFACE OF THE PLANET AND THE MAJOR COMPONENTS OF YOUR BODY IS WATER

Therefore, you should replenish your water supply daily with clean, pure water.

The next probing question is... since you are composed of approximately 85 percent water, to flourish how much of your diet should be made up of clean, pure water for replacement, and raw water-rich foods (fruits and vegetables)?

You might take a moment and think back to the last real sit down meal you had. If we were to look at the food on your plate, would we find foods that are rich in water? Would we see any foods that are in a whole, uncooked state? Might the volume of that uncooked food be 50 percent of the plate, or perhaps 30 percent ... 10 percent, or even less? For instance, if it was dinner, would we be looking at pork chops and potatoes, and a microscopic portion of an overcooked vegetable? Or, would we see a large portion of lightly steamed vegetables, a salad and a modest portion of concentrated foods (starch or meat)? Before eating, when you look at your plate, make sure you are eating more high-water-content foods, and more raw foods that contain a lot of water, vitamins, minerals, enzymes, etc., that are unheated and untampered with.

Your meals should be a mix of concentrated foods (cooked food), and high-water-content foods. What are high-water-content foods? Let me tell you first what are NOT high-water-content foods. Coffee is not, beer and wine are not, milk from cows does not count for our purposes, ("Mother's milk" for babies, however, is their perfect food). Soda pop certainly does not cut it. Bread is not, meat if eaten raw would be, but since that is dangerous, and not socially acceptable (exception for native Eskimos), we won't include it. Meat as we prepare it, barbecued, broiled, fried or microwaved, is not high in water content. In fact, most foods that are cooked or processed in any way end up as concentrated foods regardless of how water-rich they started out.

Are you beginning to get the picture? Your body needs water for replacement. The only difference between a lake and a swamp is the swamp is stagnant. A lake has a stream of "new" water flowing in all the time, while at the other end of the lake a stream of "old" water is flowing out. The continual exchange helps the lake remain fresh and clean. Meanwhile, the swamp ferments in its own waste. So do you want to be a lake or a swamp?

One last thought about consuming a large portion of your water through fruits and vegetables: There are a lot of poisons in the environment today. The root systems of these plants in the ground help to filtrate the water supplied to the plant. Some of the best sources of fluid are to be eaten (not drunk) thanks to fruits and vegetables and their root filters.

As for the water that comes directly into your body through drinking, you must realize that the toxins I mentioned a moment ago have, unfortunately, made their way into our homes. We mistakenly take for granted that the water flowing through our faucet is clean, pure and free of contaminants. Please don't assume that. So far, 819 cities, as mentioned earlier, have been found to contain unhealthy levels of one of the most obvious and toxic heavy metals ... lead. Who would ever dream that in our enlightened society people are still drinking water contaminated by lead in their own homes? But, that's not all: Pesticides and insecticides have also made it into public water systems.

Chlorine, an extremely toxic chemical, is purposely added into your water for the very reason that it kills things. Chlorine has been used very effectively in war to kill people. The water districts add chlorine to your drinking water to kill microscopic beasts, like E Coli and its friends. One could certainly make a reasonable argument that chlorination is necessary in metropolitan areas to control micro-organisms in central water districts, but that's where it ends. Chlorine should not end up in your orange juice! One could hardly make a reasonable case that after the water has safely made it from the water district to your faucet, you should go ahead and swallow a known poison. The chlorine has done its job before arriving at your house, and does not need to be in your glass! This stuff is no longer your friend. You should not be drinking chlorine, period. Can you imagine that removing chlorine from your daily diet might be, perhaps, 5 percent of the total answer to allowing your body to function properly again?

Fluoride is another interesting added substance. I have a few friends who are dentists and most (but not all) of them are fairly quick to point out the value of fluoride for stronger teeth. I acknowledge that there might be some value, and if people "choose" to brush their teeth with fluoridated toothpaste and have fluoride treatments by their dentist, that is fine. But to blindly and continually drink fluoride, a known toxin, is certainly overkill and potentially dangerous.

I was recently presenting seminars in Australia. One attendee provided me with a publication with the following reprint from the *Canberra Times*, Aug. 5, 1993. The title read...

FLUORIDE CAN DAMAGE CHILDREN'S TEETH: DENTIST

"Parents have been warned not to let their children use too much toothpaste because excess fluoride can damage their teeth. The Australian Dental Association and NSW (New South Wales) Health Department have warned that children under two should not use toothpaste at all and older children should be given children's toothpaste which has less than half the amount of fluoride of adult toothpaste. Children up to the age of seven should be supervised while brushing their teeth to prevent them swallowing the toothpaste."

The publication then goes on to criticize the Australian media for only making this information public in New South Wales, neglecting the families in other states.

The water we drink and cook with must be pure and clean, distilled if necessary. All of these additives make the water coming through your faucet a mutant of what it is supposed to be. When consumed for 10 and 20 years, or more ... what damaging (yet subtle) effects are occurring on a cellular level? We'll probably never know, except for what we see going on around us.

A simple water filtration system can eliminate a lot of these, and other contaminates, before they pass your lips. Information on water filtration systems and other products and services I recommend are contained in the back of this book.

Action Step: The water you consume needs to be pure. Water is intimately connected with the metabolic functions of your body. Remember the lake/swamp metaphor. Be a crystal clear mountain lake. Consume a lot of "new" clean water every day.

Now on to **FOOD**! Finally, we can talk about **FOOD** ... one of my favorite subjects! Not so much a favorite subject to talk about, but rather a subject of consumption ... I love to eat! *Food, not* baseball, is the great American pastime!

Here is a word of "caution & celebration"... I am not a nutritionist. I have never claimed to be one, nor will I ever. **This is actually good news for you**, because I'm not about to get into the chemistry of nutrition, but rather, I'll share some of my clinical experiences. I have gathered some data that seems to be useful. I have seen some pretty incredible results from small dietary alterations, but I never want to be considered an expert in the field of nutrition. Here's why ... The diagnosis and treatment of a condition through nutrition (although very valuable) is equal, philosophically, to treating someone with medicines. And, I don't have the ego to look at a complex organism made up of trillions of interconnected working parts (your body) and pretend that I can figure out exactly what is lacking in the workings of this marvel.

Sometimes a nutritional approach is necessary and appropriate (sometimes, on a gross level, it is obvious what is lacking), but this has little to do with amplifying your Life-force. It would be more akin to practicing medicine. Remember, we are trying to develop your deductive reasoning skills. We're still working on the big picture. Rather than just relying on doctors to tell us exactly what our bodies are deficient in (who in most cases don't even know what's going on in their own bodies), let's see if we can develop some ideas that make sense to you personally. This is about thinking for yourself and reclaiming some of your personal responsibility. I also intend for this to be easy enough so you will be inclined to _do_ what you _know_, not just to _know_ what you _know_.

We've got to avoid "popular fashion" or the "latest rage:" For instance, the popularity of Vitamin C one year, then Vitamin E the next. A few short years ago Laetrile was "the" cure for cancer, now it has apparently disappeared. I'm sure all of these materials have value, but there is so much more. Why get caught up in isolating a few components in a sea of tens of thousands of them. By the end of this year, I would wager that science will discover "new" properties in apples and broccoli that have always been there; we just now are stumbling upon unknown factors. Let's not get hung up on the few components of whole food that science is identifying.

In a layman's sort of way, I guess I am an expert in food. I have a Ph.D. in results from the school of *"try anything that makes sense."* I, perhaps like you, started out on TV dinners and canned spaghetti, thanks to the prevailing ignorance and the multimedia of the 1950s and 1960s. Then, as an athlete, I began eating large quantities of meat protein, wheat germ and potatoes and gravy.

Later in life I became a vegetarian; I really cleaned up my program. In fact, for a number of reasons I became what is referred to as a vegan for a year. A vegan Vegetarian is someone who, in addition to eating no meat, also eats no other animal products like milk, butter, and so on. I believe vegetarianism is a valid way of living. No explanation needed when one looks to a group like the Seventh Day Adventists. Statistically, as a group, these vegetarians appear to suffer from less degenerative disease and simply have longer life spans than the rest of the population. I am no longer a vegetarian, but it may be absolutely perfect for you.

I then stumbled upon "Food Combining." All of these approaches to eating have value and shortcomings. But "proper" food combining made even more sense to me. Food combining advocates claim that when we eat a starch-based food (bread, potato, rice), our body secretes alkaline digestive juices in order to properly digest that starchy type of food. And, when we eat a protein-based food (most commonly meats), the stomach secretes acid digestive juices in order to properly utilize that type of food. These secretions are commonly understood in the nutritional and scientific community, and are agreed-upon observations.

The interesting part comes when we combine both carbohydrates (starch) and protein in our meals at the one sitting. You don't need to be a chemist to know that when an alkaline is combined with an acid the two will cancel each other out. If an acid and a base are mixed ... they will neutralize each other. So, if you eat a piece of chicken and then have a bowl of rice, in theory, you are telling your body to produce both acid and alkaline digestive juices simultaneously. They, of course, would then cancel each other out (if mixed), resulting in incomplete and ineffective digestion of your meal. If this is true (and I can't say that it is for everyone, since we are "individuals"), the protein would putrefy and the starches would ferment in your gut.

Here's a great example of miscombining a meal, and I'm sure someone reading this book has done this. Let's just imagine you go to your local fast food franchise for lunch. You order a <u>hamburger</u>, a <u>milk shake</u> and a bag of <u>fries</u>. The protein and starch, as mentioned, do not combine well, throw in the grease and the dairy, and your lunch is a real mess. Although "filling," these foods slow your blood stream and stress your nervous system. You go back to work feeling full but lethargic, like you need a nap. Rather than **extracting** energy from the foods you ate, your body is now **expending** energy just trying to digest and push them through the gut for elimination. Since eating this way often causes energy depletion, you may feel tired and lethargic after eating. Indigestion and gas may also be an indication that you are experiencing incomplete digestion of your meals.

Food combining advocates suggest centering your meals around *either* starch or proteins and avoid combining the two in the same meal. For instance ... a dinner could be centered around meat, if that's what you want, and it might include a nice salad and some steamed vegetables. If you didn't want to have meat for a particular meal, then try the same steamed veggies, a big salad and a big baked potato with all the trimmings (except bacon bits!). The main theme to food combining is to avoid mixing starches and proteins, which seems to make sense. But we're all so different. I've met some people who have lived long, healthy lives and broken every rule that food combining (and vegetarianism) might suggest, without noticeable intestinal distress or other noticeable short comings. Apparently, they had other Foundational Keys engaged, supplying surplus power and nerve energy to over-ride these less empowering habits.

There are other rules to food combining that make sense, like eating fruits only on an empty stomach. Why does that make sense? Because fruits are digested in the intestines, not the stomach. If eaten properly, fruit spends very little time in the stomach. So, if you eat fruit after a typical meal, the fruit will get stuck in your stomach behind the starches and/or protein, which need to spend a fair amount of time in the stomach. Fruit should only land in the stomach for a few minutes. After that, I'm told by food combiners, it begins to decay and ferment.

Food combining can't hurt you. It probably isn't "the" total answer for you, but give it a try, particularly if you are trying to regain some portion of your energy. Imagine trying to regain your health, yet losing 20-30 percent of your healing nerve energy to in-effective and overstressed digestive processes because of the way you are eating. It's being wasted on trying to separate out your foods and then pushing this "material" through the digestive tract. In the all-out effort to amplify and regain your health, do try food combining with a fair amount of discipline as an effort to conserve the healing energy available to you.

READERS WHO ARE WELL, AND THOSE WHO ARE ALSO INTERESTED IN LONGEVITY AND PEAK PERFORMANCE ... TAKE HEED OF THESE WORDS ON FOOD COMBINING AND NUTRITION.

Practically speaking, we all miscombine meals and "deductively," I know the body can handle it most of the time. Let's just be aware of this concept, and wisely use this data as you see appropriate.

Food combining makes good sense. Yet I don't have the discipline to do it all the time, nor do I believe a healthy person must do it continually, **IF** he or she will recognize and live according to this next very important concept.

Here, now, is the one nutritional *"must"* that **CANNOT BE COMPROMISED.** There is really no controversy on this section, so we will need to be in complete agreement.

You need to eat a lot of living, unadulterated, unprocessed whole foods. Eat foods that have *not* been canned, fried, microwaved, cooked or heated. I'm talking about raw foods. I'm talking about live foods. In particular, I'm talking about **raw** fruits and vegetables.

First of all, why fruits and vegetables? Because they are the *perfect* foods. They contain all the vitamins we've been talking about all these years and they have the minerals, too. When you buy those bottles of fragmented vitamins, i.e. Vitamin C, E, and even those multivitamin pills ... where do you think the manufacturer gets his selected vitamins? Fruits and Vegetables, of course! Fruits and Vegetables are easy to digest, there is no cholesterol and little fat (the fat that is present is far more friendly to your body than animal fat).

Recently, we've heard from the media all about something called phyto-chemicals. Phyto means plant. These are chemicals that are found only in plants (like fruits and vegetables). Five years ago we didn't know they existed. I'd never heard of Phytochemicals. Science is now learning that phyto-chemicals are incredibly beneficial to human health, yet, they are only beginning to identify the many thousands of them. These chemicals have always existed, but "man" has just begun to scratch the surface. There may be tens of thousands of chemicals and elements that allow a carrot, to be a carrot. In light of this, you may begin to understand how the bottles of vitamins you have purchased in the past offer only a small identified sliver of the complete nutrition we're all looking for. Solution ... go back to the source, volumes of whole uncooked fruits and vegetables.

Science continues to discover some of the pieces to the puzzle. Yet, in the next decade they may find ten thousand more elements which are now unnamed and unknown, but all beneficial and necessary for life. I recently had a patient tell me that he was participating in a research project at the famous Fred Hutchinson Cancer Center. He was on a prescribed dose of carotene, an enzyme from carrots. He informed me that "they" believed this fragment of the carrot holds a strong possible link to curing and/or preventing cancer. Do you see the folly with that line of thinking? Sure carotene is important, but don't they think God put the carrot together as a package deal? (**Post script:** *the research project was scrapped as the test results were coming out very unfavorable. In this test the imbalanced, increased beta carotene dosages actually <u>advanced</u> cancer growth in some patients. Again, I say it's the whole food not the individual components.*)

The cure for conditions from A to Z is not likely to be found in one fragment of a carrot or the bark of the yew tree. Nor, as in the early 1970s, when I was taught that we (the U.S.A.) had scientific teams in submarines under the polar ice caps looking for the cure to cancer on the under belly of the unborn fetus of a white whale! Perhaps that sounds absurd today, but what will our children think in 25 years about what we call science. I'm sure there are a lot of Beluga Whales under the polar ice caps that are happy we gave up that witch hunt!

The point is, whole food is a **key** to whole health. Nature (God, if I may) is perfect, we will never harness it, so we must learn to work *with* the natural process and, in doing so, amplify the Life-force. Again, I feel I should clarify that this book, while focused on helping headache sufferers, is not about curing one disease or another. The purpose of this book is to help you amplify the potential you already have. I would like to help you achieve the healing and help you stay well, so you won't need pills, potions or the bark of the yew tree.

So, what is it about whole raw foods that is so great? The answer ... *"Nothing, and yet everything."* Whole foods are not mysterious until science breaks them down into tiny pieces (inductively), then gives the tiny pieces names which only scientists can pronounce. That's how things in the health world get confusing! Whole foods are normal, they are what we are supposed to eat. Whole foods contain the necessary stuff of life. Our departure from nature is usually what gets us into trouble. Our habits of overcooking, boiling, frying, chemically preserving and now microwaving, destroy the normalcy inherent in whole food.

So, to state it another way, whole foods are the only complete foods. We need to recognize how invalid processed foods are, since they so frequently end up on our plates.

One of the most important characteristics of a whole food, and yet, the first component to be destroyed in heating/processing, is the inherent enzymes. What is an enzyme? To paraphrase *Webster's Dictionary*, *"enzymes are protein-like substances that act as catalysts in initiating or speeding up chemical reactions (in your body) and usually become inactive and unstable at high temperatures."* Even *Webster's* knew we're messing things up when we cook so much of our food!

For our purposes, there are only two general types of enzymes, <u>dietary</u> and <u>metabolic</u>. Dietary enzymes are the necessary enzymes you obtain from raw fruits and vegetables. Metabolic enzymes are inherent within your body. They are used to facilitate nearly all of the metabolic functions going on inside at any given time. Without enzymes life would not be possible. Your metabolic enzymes are limited in quantity, somewhat like a bank account. If you supply your body with plenty of dietary enzymes, you will be making "deposits" into your metabolic enzyme account. If not enough dietary enzymes are provided, the body will begin making "withdrawals" from its metabolic bank account. Your body is able, for a time, to "lend" enzymes from its own account. But the body eventually demands repayment, via dietary enzymes. Many of the people I consult with are, enzymatically speaking, "overdrawn."

The condition of the enzymes is said to be what makes a food "alive" or "dead." There is a very simple test you can run at home to find out the state of the enzymes in your foods. Let me explain, if you were to gather some beans, peas, or alfalfa seeds from your garden, steam half the seeds for just a minute or two, plant those same seeds in the ground (or a sprouting container) and water them, I would suggest they would not sprout because there is no longer any life; the enzymes are denatured, inactivated.....dead. Take the remaining seeds or peas, skip the cooking part of the experiment and plant them the same way. Can you guess what will occur? Of course! The uncooked peas will sprout and grow because that's what they are designed to do. They still have that mysterious power of life in them. Incidentally, just adding water to alfalfa seeds increases the nutritional value by up to 300 percent.

Eating denatured enzymes ... cooked food -is like eating dead food. We all do it, and I'm not suggesting we throw out our pots and pans! I am suggesting that we make a conscious effort to ingest much more food with "live" (active) enzymes.

As mentioned earlier, the Cancer Society and the Heart Foundation have come out publicly to aggressively endorse the practice of eating five or more servings of raw fruits and five servings of raw vegetables **everyday.** Now, come on, that's a lot of produce! Yet, that's what they're saying each one of us needs to do to avoid catastrophic diseases. Did you have your five servings of raw fruits and vegetables today? Do you remember the last time you did? Have you ever had that much raw produce in one day? Wow! Just imagine how your health might benefit immediately, and in the future, if for the next six months you added to your present diet the volumes they are suggesting.

When you were born, you were issued a "Bank Account" of metabolic enzymes. These are your enzymes that your body needs to keep things running smoothly. Hopefully, your mother had the good sense, and ability, to breastfeed you, supplying you with even more of these vital enzymes (mommy's milk is alive and complete, unlike baby formulas and even pasteurized milk). So, mom was helping you make "bank deposits" early on. And a good thing, too. If you're like me, the eating habits of your early years led you to as much over-cooked-dead, greasy processed food as you could possibly find.

If you continue eating enzyme deficient foods, then your body will need to borrow from your ever-decreasing "private" (metabolic) enzyme account. Your body expects you to pay back your enzyme debt. Yet, more often than not, we continue eating processed foods and keep borrowing and borrowing against our personal metabolic enzyme account. I hope you are way ahead of so many Americans who on average spend less than $2.00 per week in the produce department of the grocery store. According to the University of California Medical School, the three most commonly eaten foods in the United States are white bread, coffee, and hot dogs. Every year the typical American eats 23 gallons of ice cream, 7 pounds of potato chips, 365 servings of soda pop, 90 pounds of fat, and 134 pounds of refined sugar! In the case of these "typical" Americans (who unknowingly suffer from a lack of dietary enzymes), their own "private bank account" of enzymes are initially borrowed from the skeleton causing osteoporosis, for starters. If continued, enzymes are taken from more vital internal organs. Later on, the body just doesn't have what it is entitled to (or needs) for normal function. It is still waiting for you to repay your enzyme debt. Therefore, a breakdown has to occur somewhere, often in the immune system. This scenario contributes to an increase stress load on your body. Do you think a lack of phytochemicals and dietary enzymes could be another significant contributor to your headache problems? If you're not getting active enzymes into your diet, it could be another portion of your complete headache answer.

Enzymes are incredibly important. A research project back in the 1940s demonstrated the importance of dietary enzymes. This is the first study I know of where medical science documented and looked at the value of processed foods and the benefits of dietary enzymes. In other words, the question was asked, *"Do processed foods affect our well- being?"* This landmark project was done by a Dr. Pottinger, a medical doctor. It's important to know that this doctor was not financed by the dairy industry or the cattle industry-he financed his own research. So nobody was telling him what to do, or what results to expect. He just wanted to know if the consumption of processed foods would affect mammals.

Cats were his experimental animals. He took approximately 900 cats and divided them into two groups. He fed only live food to one group: meat, vegetables, and so on , not cooked or processed. The other group he fed processed food. He was trying to determine any differences. He found, of course, that the "live food" cats, did fine. They lived a normal cat life span, approximately 14 to 16 years. But, he found that the "processed food cats" in their later years, developed health problems. Not only flus, colds and sore throats, but cancer, diabetes and chronic degenerative diseases; illnesses we often see in our elderly and sometimes our young people, too.

The second generation of "processed food cats" also showed up with chronically degenerative diseases. But, rather than occuring at the end of their life span, these diseases tended to show up about midway through their life as arthritis, diabetes, cancer and so on. The third generation of "processed food cats" started to show the same chronic degenerative diseases in kittenhood. Some were born with chronic diseases. Many of them developed chronic degenerative diseases within the first month or two of their life and did not live a full life span. The third generation became sick very early. It is also interesting to note that the third generation could not reproduce. They were not able to bear offspring. This forced the end of the research project. Meanwhile, the second and third generations of "whole food cats" continued to live normal cat lifespans. We (our society) are in the third and forth generations of offspring since our grand parents and great-grand parents left the farm and were introduced to convenient canned and otherwise processed foods. I believe, without a shadow of a doubt, that even with all the nutritional information available, there are more nutrient-based health problems occuring today due, in part, by poor choices made by today's consumer. But, some of the problems may well stem from processed food consumption by mom and dad, grandpa and grandma.

I'm certain you realize that food and water are significant keys to health. Yet, few of us would be willing to eat five or more servings of raw fruits and vegetables every day and **continue** doing it regardless of the inconvenience. Someone once told me that people are more likely to change their religion than their eating habits!

I personally bought a juicer a few years ago to juice large amounts of produce and get all the nutrition I had been missing. But, after a few short weeks our new juicer found its way to the dark recesses of our pantry floor, seldom to be heard from again. Juicing is a great idea but for us it was simply too messy, too time-consuming and rather expensive.

TWO TYPES OF FOOD -- LIVE AND DEAD

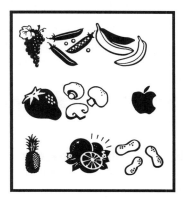 

In school we're taught all about the different food groups (proteins, fats, etc.), but I see a greater distinction, for our purposes, by simplifying our classifications into two food groups: "live" foods, and foods that are "dead," inactivated by processing. One of the most vital bits of information you can pull from this chapter and act on immediately, is to know that if the food is raw or uncooked you will gain more benefits (excluding certain animal products) than ingesting the same food cooked.

Eating foods rich in "live" enzymes also helps us digest our foods. All food taken into the body must be broken down into smaller units in the digestive tract to be utilized by the body. This breaking down process is done largely by enzymes. If the consumed food is enzyme deficient, then, as you can probably guess, your body has to pitch in and lend more of its own metabolic enzyme supply, using more energy and adding greater stress to the body. If, however, the food is enzyme rich, these consumed enzymes significantly aid in the digestive process, and you will be making "deposits" to your own enzyme "bank account." Enzymes in raw foods help the digestive process up to 75 percent, without the need for metabolic enzymes secreted by the body. Wow- what a great return on your investment! All that energy saved can be used in other beneficial ways to advance your healing processes, improve your longevity and clear your head of pain.

But are you going to eat five (or more) servings of fresh raw fruit and vegetables every day? That's really a lot when you consider how little time and money the average American spends in the produce department per week.

Now, you may get really motivated and eat properly for a few days, or even a couple of weeks. However, old patterns and habits usually kick in eventually, overriding these good intentions. Or perhaps your family will rebel and eat at a restaurant, without inviting you!

Because so many people are accustomed to eating processed foods, many have lost their taste for raw fruits and vegetables. And many people simply don't want to change their habits. They like the food they eat because it provides social value, personal entertainment and fulfillment.

Therefore, I won't try to change your dietary habits. If you

are eating volumes of raw fruits and vegetables each day, con-
gratulations and keep it up! If, like me, you are a little
shy of five servings of each every day, or if you never touch
the stuff ... I do have good news for you, too, and you <u>don't</u>
have to change!

There are a precious few products available on the market
that actually supplement the whole food benefits of fruits
and vegetables. I've found one product that supplies significant amounts of enzymes and phytochemicals by simply
swallowing four capsules of concentrated fruit and vegetable
material each day with water.

Just imagine how your health could benefit if you were to
consume the equivalent of nearly 300 pounds of raw produce each month for the next year! And, this can be done
without really changing your eating habits! It would be a
great investment for not only your present health, but towards your future and your children's future, also. If you
are not going to consume five to nine servings of raw fruits
and raw vegetables on an on-going daily basis, this is your
next best source. Please consult the back of this book for
product information that could fulfill your nutritional needs.

Action Steps: Our health would benefit from a return to
the land. Since that isn't likely to occur, we need to eat in a
way that is compatible and supportive with the design and needs
of our body. Increase your intake of *clean* water. Food
combining is a worthy consideration. Try to eat less starches
and proteins in the same meal. Raw "live" foods contain
phytochemicals and "live" enzymes. Enzymes are over-looked,
yet incredibly important. Five servings of raw fruits and raw
vegetables are now considered a minimum. If you don't have

the discipline to follow through, or simply can't afford the time and need something more convenient (than cutting and cleaning vegetables all day), consult the back of the book for a supplemental product that can fill the void between what you need and what you are getting. Proper nutrition is incredibly important to eliminating headache, and fending off "normal" decay and degenerative diseases associated with our "civilized " lifestyle and processed food consumption.

Putting out the fire in your head is significantly assisted by stoking the fire in your body, but we'll only warm you up for starters. Let's not overdo this because it needs to be fun!

I completely endorse a slow but steady introduction to......

• Chapter Nine •

EXERCISE
Foundational Key *#3*

"The dictionary is the only place where success comes before work."
--Mark Twain

What can I possibly say about the virtues of exercise that you haven't already heard a thousand times? What can I show you about exercise that you haven't already tried? Most middle-income Americans have at least two exercise contraptions in their homes, purchased with every good intention. And as you know (perhaps personally), the vast majority of them are collecting dust, out of sight... in the corner or the closet.

These words on exercise, however, will be different. These words will not fall on deaf ears because this is not about losing a beer belly or saddle bags. We'll only look at exercise as either a Foundational Key blocking your way to using more of your Life-force, or as an activity you regularly enjoy.

Again, this is not about weight loss ... but rather, a system to oxygenate your blood stream. Headache sufferers nearly always benefit from exercise, and as you continue to participate in the enjoyable activities *you* have chosen, you may very well notice some "poundage" dropping off as a side benefit. In the early 1960s, President John F. Kennedy clearly stated that we are a society of spectators. Little has changed in 40 years. Now we have a cute name for men who sit all weekend watching sports on TV ... are there any *"Couch Potatoes"* in your family?

the fan by John McPherson

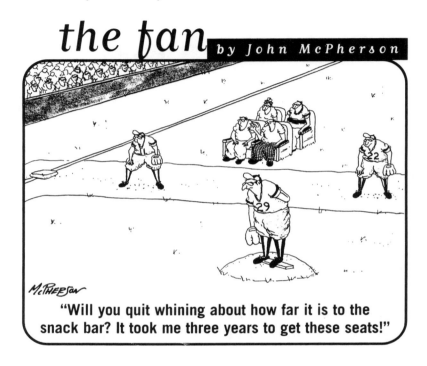

"Will you quit whining about how far it is to the snack bar? It took me three years to get these seats!"

I'm not going to tell you what you need to do. In fact, I don't know what you specifically need to do as far as exercising *your* body. If I told you to go and peddle a bicycle for three miles every day, perhaps you might do it for a while, but because you didn't choose it yourself ... you wouldn't be committed to staying with it for any length of time. Instead, find something that is physical, that you'd like to do.   Strive to eventually get your pulse rate elevated for 20 or 30 minutes, three times per week. Don't let yourself get winded. Exercise in such a way that you can still carry on a conversation, but definitely feel yourself warming up during the workout time. Initially, you may only be able to carry out your activity for five minutes. Later on, if you can do more activities, such as weight lifting, racketball, a team sport, or whatever, that's great -- *just keep at it!*

Oh, yes, a message from my attorney: ***If you have a health condition that you feel may be complicated by exercising, please consult your physician before starting.*** With that said, and my legal responsibility to my family fulfilled, I would like to add that I believe there are few situations where some form of exercise or movement would not be beneficial. Even if the patient is flat on his or her back, some sort of movement is vital to assist the body in pumping the lymph (garbage transport) system.

Patients who are inactive often compound their problem by not getting any form of movement. Decreased oxygenation occurs. Stagnation of the body fluids sets in, the toxic environment builds up, and the patient, ultimately, has less and less desire to get moving. I see a fair number of people "diagnosed" with Chronic Fatigue Syndrome. What would you guess that 90 percent of these people, whom I've consulted, have in common? Chronic Inactivity. I know that the more inactive I am, the less I want to become active ... I become more fatigued by the less I do! There are certainly other considerations, but my observation is that most of these people slowed down

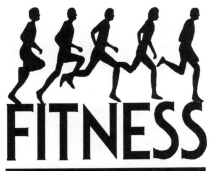

long before the Chronic Fatigue became a syndrome. In physiology, there is a concept that, "What you don't use ... you'll lose." In physics it's called "inertia," a body in motion tends to stay in motion ... and conversely, a body at rest tends to stay at rest.

The human body is a lot like nature in some ways. As I mentioned earlier, the water content of the body corresponds pretty much to the percentage of water on the planet. But in some ways the body is very different from nature. For instance, the more natural resources we pull out of the earth the less there are. Eventually we will drain the vast supply of minerals and fossil fuels. But your body is the opposite, the more you use your body, the stronger it gets. The more you use any part of your body, within reason, the better it gets. The more you read, or engage in stimulating conversation, the better the brain cell connections become. If you are an artist, more painting will improve your nerve connections for that activity. If you play golf, the more you play, more neuro-connections will actually grow for the purpose of making you a better golfer. If you are a mathematician, and you study math several hours per day, the same thing happens, you'll grow more connections for math! This process is called "neuroplasticity." Neuroplasticity ensures biologically that we all become better at whatever we do the most. It is literally the growing of nerve pathways within the brain that allows us to excel at our most frequented activities. Unfortunately, if children watch hours of MTV, and that's where their interests lie, then that's what they become good at. Walking, rowing, swimming, bike riding, weight lifting, whatever you decide, even for the bedridden patient, the more you do it, the stronger and more vital you will become.

Your body is a gift- the Bible refers to it as a temple ... even the greatest temples need some house cleaning, so get moving and take care of your gift.

Here is a special bonus to those readers who are becoming somewhat   overwhelmed with these six little Foundational Keys. Perhaps you noticed that if you turn this key, and stay with it, you will be oxygenating your body automatically. You'll also be pumping the lymph to help activate garbage removal in the blood stream. What a great deal! If you exercise, you won't have to think about **Foundational Key #1, AIR** — it's handled, compliments of **Foundational Key #3 — EXERCISE**.

Action Step: I won't tell you <u>what</u> to do. Just find a physical activity you can enjoy and will stay with, figure out when and where you're going to do it, then get started. You might be wondering, *does he want me to exercise <u>when</u> I have a headache?* The answer is, you probably won't enjoy yourself. Peddling a bicycle with a splitting headache would not be fun, and you won't continue unless you're having a good time. It would be best not to start under those circumstances.

It's hard to believe that this next subject could be an obstacle for people. This Foundational Key consumes one third of your life. That would be 30 years if you only live to be 90. It is incredibly important in the scheme of your life, and since you'll spend so much time doing it, let's not take it for granted. I'm talking about ways to get more benefits out of ......

• Chapter Ten •

SLEEP
Foundational Key *#4*

How long do you believe the human body was built to last? Physiologists tell me that this body was designed to live at least 120 to 170 years! But if you last "only" 90 years you will most likely sleep an accumulated 30 years of your lifetime away. That would be 1/3 of your life, approximately eight hours each day. But sleeping certainly is not a waste of time.

Have you ever slept a headache away? How does that happen? When you sleep, the brain changes its physiological state. In layman's terms, you're taking the edge off. A good night's sleep disengages the "live ammunition" that could have triggered a headache.

While you sleep you are recharging your batteries. Your body is rebuilding itself on the cellular level. Patients with headaches sometimes find it difficult to sleep, and conversely, patients with insomnia are prone to have more headaches. Which came first, the chicken or the egg? Answer ... it really doesn't matter, what counts is working with the cause and reestablishing a balance in the person's life.

Prolonged loss of sleep is associated with progressive malfunction of the mind and activities of the nervous system. Surely you have noticed the increased sluggishness of thought and irritability occurring toward the end of extended hours without sleep. Patients can even become psychotic following forced periods of prolonged wakefulness. Sleep somehow, although not well understood, balances out the needs of the physical body, the nervous system, and the Life-force!

Since sleep is so important, it makes sense that we should learn how to best support our bodies while sleeping to get the most out of this rebuilding time.

1) *Be sure to have a supportive mattress.* What exactly does that mean?   Well, to some people it means a waterbed. I slept on a waterbed for over 12 years and for much of that time I recommended it to everyone. I was truly dedicated to waterbeds. In my opinion they were warm and comfortable. However, after convincing one man, who was large enough to play linebacker on any NFL team, to purchase one, I was cured of telling people only to purchase waterbeds. Not long after his purchase he decided he didn't care for his new waterbed, and the company he bought it from didn't want to honor his return agreement. At one point, I thought he was going to feed me his bed. It all worked out in the long run. He eventually got a suitable bed and I learned two important lessons:

      A. Always give people choices.
      B. We are all different and have unique needs
      (from bedding to nutrition), for we are all constantly changing and adapting.

I said I slept on waterbeds for twelve years. I really enjoyed those beds. But during the last year or so my spine and muscles were changing. I can't say exactly how, but both my wife and I were not as refreshed in the morning as before. We experimented with different water levels but to no avail.

We did some market research, which included a bit of reading and a lot of jumping on, and lying on, display beds in stores. We then ordered what we felt was the best value and support system on the market today. After three years we both agree there is no turning back. We are extremely happy with the new, more conventional bed.

Whatever you decide, make sure your spine is well-supported. I had one patient who I knew should be getting better results from my care and instructions than he was reporting to me. I began to question him about different things he might be doing that were counter productive to our desired results. When we got to bedding, I asked him what kind of mattress he slept on. He said, "Oh, I've got a great bed, Doc. It's 20 years old, shaped like a bowl and when I lie down on it, it wraps right around me like a canoe. I love that bed!" Well, we got him out of that bed, and after a couple of weeks of getting used to his new mattress, he was on the mend. I now recommend to my patients and clients that they consider a new bed every five to 10 years, or at a maximum 10 to 15 years.

2) ***Sleep on your back or your side.*** Literally hundreds of times in my practice I've had patients in as near perfect balance as could be obtained. They had been doing fine, no headaches for months and even years in some cases, only to find that they apparently had slept in a twisted position, unraveling a perfect correction. Most importantly, the neck needs to remain in a relaxed, neutral position. Sleeping on your stomach for eight hours every night is a sure way to tangle up the nerves and muscles in your neck. Stomach sleeping is allowed only if I can come to your home and cut a hole out of your mattress so you can look straight down towards the floor. When you sleep on your stomach you are twisting your neck, closing off vital nerve pathways. Okay, I know, you've been sleeping this way for as long as you can

remember. I also know that sleeping on one's stomach is a very difficult pattern to break. But consider what twisting your neck for eight hours each night, for 30 years of your life, might do. This just may be a significant contributing factor to insufficient neurological supply, causing anything from migraine headaches to immune disorders. The position of your neck vertebrae is quite important when considering your well-being and recovery. Since we're talking about 1/3 of your lifetime, let's learn to sleep correctly, and not scrimp on proper support.

When you sleep on your back your pillow should support your head and neck, not force it forward. Stand with your back to a wall, with your heels against the wall, and notice the distance between your neck and head, and the wall. This would provide a good measurement for most people when determining how thick their pillow should be.

If you sleep on your side, put your shoulder to the wall and measure the width between the wall and your head. That's how thick your pillow should be if you are a side-posture sleeper.

You'll notice that in both instances the head and neck end up in a neutral relaxed position. Neither bent forward, bent backwards, or twisted. That is how we need to sleep, in as "neutral" a position as possible for the neck and spine.

This question comes up frequently: "What if I twist around into different positions during the night?" No worries, just ask yourself to flatten the pillow out for sleeping on your back and bunch it up for sleeping on your side. Your "subconscious" mind will respond and serve your best interests. Just as army personnel can be trained to sleep with their eyes open, you can learn to adjust your pillow for changing postures. I

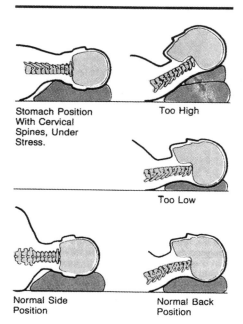

Stomach Position With Cervical Spines, Under Stress.

Too High

Too Low

Normal Side Position

Normal Back Position

sleep with a well-filled feather pillow. It conforms easily to the different sleeping postures I acquire during the night. You can learn to do the same.

The whole idea behind sleeping is to wake up refreshed and ready to go. Many people with whom I consult tell me they "wake up tired" and have been getting up in the morning for the last 10 to 20 years with no energy. I would say to you, at this point, if you are someone who wakes up without much energy as often as two or three times per week, then you should consider this symptom a warning that your health may be taking a turn for the worse in the not-too-distant future.

As mentioned earlier, some of these ideas may initially seem trivial but may be incredibly vital to your recovery. Therefore, please read and reread this book, then apply to your lifestyle as much of the information and techniques as you see fit.

Frequently, people will try to justify their lack of energy by saying or thinking they are just getting older. But I would submit there are 65 -and 70-year-old people waking up every morning with energy and vital bodies. I've attempted to learn from both groups of people, those who suffer through life, and those who have lived long, productive lives with energy and vibrant bodies. I've decided to pattern my life after the second set of habits (you can decide to do that, too). I also want to learn from people who have destroyed their health, and avoid as many of the common habits of this group as I can identify. In essence, that is what I have done with this book, shared with you in a boiled down version.

People who are unable to sleep (insomniacs) are individuals who desperately need sleep. Have you ever been awake for 36 or 48 hours, and for a while you're even too tired to sleep? That gives you a little taste of what chronic insomnia is like. Invariably, insomniacs are out of sync with the needs of their bodies. In most of these cases, a modest adjustment to one or two of the Foundational Keys to health will restore a more normal sleeping pattern.

Action Steps: You are going to sleep 30 years of your life away -it is the part of the day that your cells are recharging. Do it wisely. Don't cut corners. If the bed is worn out ... just like those $120 tennis shoes we get for the kids, throw it out when the time comes. Sleep on your back or on your side, with a modest sized pillow ... Sweet dreams.

Now, you are ready for the 5th Foundational Key to living without headache pain. The initials are PMA - can you guess what it stands for?

• Chapter Eleven •

POSITIVE MENTAL ATTITUDE
Foundational Key *#5*

"Comedy is tragedy -- plus time."
--Carol Burnett

PMA, **Positive Mental Attitude**, and belief systems. Please don't misunderstand ... I'm not about to tell you that you can wish your headache gone forever with positive thinking. But what I know for certain is that a positive state of mind will enhance all that you set out in do in life. I'm proud of you ... I don't believe you would have read this far if you had a negative attitude about your future, or about this material.

Have you ever heard of Leo Buscaglia? Leo tells a wonderful story about a woman whose boss gets a speeding ticket on his way to work one morning. By the time he finally arrives, after the long delay with the officer and the yet undetermined expense of the ticket, he is really ticked off. He proceeds to take his negative state-of-mind out on his secretary once he arrives at the office. "Haven't you got this typing done yet," he bellows. "It was supposed to be done and out of here last week!"

This and other stressful encounters cause her to become increasingly angry as the day wears on. She nearly gets in an automobile accident on her way home from work. Fuming, when she finally gets home she sees that her son has torn a hole in his new trousers. This adds to her tension and causes her to explode at her son. "Those are your Sunday best, and

I told you not to wear them for play! You get to your room, and stay there."

Her son, mumbling to himself, lower lip curled over and head down, kicks the dog on his way to his room. The dog, angry and in pain, runs out of the way of further danger into the living room where he bites the cat. In a final and fitting ending to this unfortunate sequence of events that began with a speeding ticket, the cat urinates on the rug! Of course, the urine spot on the rug provides a lasting reminder of that eventful day. This story illustrates how we can let a succession of events control our attitudes. Any one of the three people could have broken the chain of events, taken a deep breath and said to him or herself, "Okay, we're off to a rough start, he's had a bad day, but there is some good in all this and I'll find out what it is later." That would have been "responding" to the situation which is positive and productive. But all three characters "reacted" to each other. A reaction is like a kneejerk action that <u>occurs without thought</u>. It is usually less useful and less productive than a response. Reactions tend to tear down bridges (in relationships), where responses tend to build bridges. Reactions tend to fuel headaches, while responses tend to calm.

Blaise Pascal, the 17th century mathematician and philosopher, wrote, *"It's not what people do to you, it's what you do with what people do to you."*

Eleanor Roosevelt more recently said, *"No one can make you feel inferior without your permission."* How true. We often give away our power and react in the negative, instead of responding positively. Something good can come from anything. Even chronic headache can provide favorable opportunities if one is looking.

Your belief systems, or your positive mental attitude, could be the topic of an entire book or a weekend seminar. It's important that you are aware of the concept because people who heal from disease and people who stay well seem to have a good mental attitude. Physiologically, if you have a negative attitude, your body is incapable of producing a substance called interferon. Perhaps you've heard of it. If a person is unfortunate enough to have cancer, the medical profession may inject interferon into the bloodstream to help fight the cancer. However, if you're talking to yourself nicely, getting along with yourself internally, if you like yourself, then your body will produce interferon naturally. The point here is that a Positive Mental Attitude is not just some fluffy, rah-rah hype, it's actually a proven physiological benefit that says if you can keep your mind right, your body will be more resilient.

Many years ago, there was a book written by Norman Cousins entitled *Anatomy of an Illness*. In his book, Mr. Cousins told his own story of how he had contracted a very serious disease. The medical community told him that he was going to die. Mr. Cousins took the diagnosis and said, "What can I do to help myself get out of this fix?" He happened to be a friend of Alan Funt, the creator of the television series "Candid Camera" in the late 1960s and early70s. So, Mr. Cousins "responded" to his condition by watching Mr. Funt's, and other comedians', television reruns which forced him to laugh, creating a positive state of mind. Even if it was a contrived laugh, by making himself do so he changed his body chemistry. He recovered from his disease, to the amazement of his doctors. Rather than lying down and dying, he made a plan *(to change his body chemistry through happiness)*, followed through with his plan, and claimed to have laughed himself back to health.

It has been observed that in every disease known to humankind, there have been people who have recovered without intervention, even from decades of continuous headaches. I spoke with a young man in Florida who was down with the final stages of cancer, a secondary result of AIDS. He had lost 50 percent of his body weight. He had a type of brain tumor that provided a very grim prognosis. He was sent home to be with his family when he died. Yet, he was suddenly able to turn his disease around and has now been in remission for years. He doesn't know how it happened. He had no particular plan to follow, except that he was strong-minded about getting the most of each day, even at 75 pounds and with no energy. There have been people with tuberculosis, cancer, heart disease, any disease that you can name, who have recovered from their disease without intervention. My belief system has always told me, and results like these confirm, that a <u>Positive Mental Attitude</u> is a major factor in many people's recovery. Don't underestimate a positive frame of mind. Rather, ask yourself what you can do to increase your happiness and laughter. Can you establish (or maintain) a bright overall outlook while you recover from chronic headaches? It might happen faster if you do, and I know you'll have more fun in the process.

Doctors often refer to these recoveries as spontaneous remissions. I'm not sure that these healings are just remissions, and I also question the term "spontaneous." Just like opening a bank vault, the tumblers must sequentially fall into place in order to get inside of that vault. The door simply won't open unless certain events occur. Although it may seem spontaneous from our viewpoint, there is nothing spontaneo us about thousands of such remissions. Certain events must occur, perhaps on a spiritual plain with one person, and a cellular/hormonal level with the next. You might think you'll be happy <u>*when*</u> the headaches leave, but perhaps the headaches will leave when you decide to be happy. Your positive mental attitude is requested for a full recovery-please comply.

One last thought on Positive Mental Attitudes: In recent years, major university medical schools, such as UCLA, have been conducting experiments to observe if positive emotions can favorably effect the body, particularly the immune system. The findings have been dramatically positive.

This approach has resulted in the development of a whole new field in medicine now called Psychoneuroimmunology (psycho-neuro-immunology). This impressive name refers to the interaction of the brain, the endocrine (hormonal) system and the immune system. Is mainstream medicine finally finding a mind/body connection to wellness? The answer seems to be a resounding ... YES!

Action Steps: We truly could get lost in this subject. Know that a positive state of mind can indeed influence your body in untold ways. Think good thoughts. See the lighter side of life and its challenges. Adopt empowering belief systems. And believe that all things happen for a reason and they serve us.

Now let's look at the undisputed champion, yet the most over looked, and least understood system of the human or-

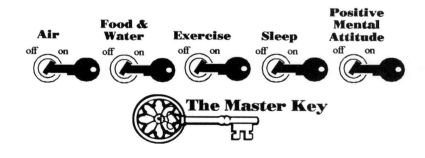

ganism. It is this system that, when out of balance, will override the other keys to health. It is this area which is, incidentally, my area of expertise. If we ever meet you'd soon realize that I spend about 90 percent of my efforts in synchronizing and engaging this master key. I'm talking about your personal "Information Super Highway," the system that carries the Life-force ...

• Chapter Twelve •

HEALTHY NERVE SYSTEM
Foundational Key #6
The Master Key

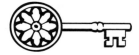

Finally, let's look at the factor that pulls the whole program together, the factor that is most overlooked, least understood, and yet, the most important: The brain and the spinal cord.

When the brain and spinal cord are not synchronized all other attempts at recovery pale they become impotent. Conversely, when the brain and nerve system are intact and working together harmoniously, all other efforts at recovery work better, nutrition is absorbed better, you'll sleep better more energy is available for activities. In fact, often times the only foundational key to health that is not engaged ... is this master key of the brain and spinal cord. Once it is properly connected, our chronic headache sufferers often see dramatic improvement on that key alone.

The brain is comprised of three sections. First, the cerebral hemispheres. That's the large part of the brain that many people think of as "the brain." But it's just the part of the brain that allows you to reason, have voluntary movement, language, knowledge, calculation and education. This area is an open book when we are born-initially it knew nothing. The cerebral portion of the brain accumulates a bit of knowledge over the years. This part of the brain may even get a degree from college and become very knowledgeable about some aspect of our world. Below and behind it is the second section, the cerebellum. The cerebellum controls fine muscle movement, balance, and coordination. It allows you to dance, skip rope and do such things as smile or write a letter to a friend. And, third, there is the brain stem. This is the area having to do with basic drives. such as appetite, anger and pleasure, sexual functions . Interestingly, it also involves tissue, organ and immune system functions. As an organized living being attempting to recover, this area of the brain is incredibly vital. It's like the switchboard between the brain and the body. The brain stem has a great deal of influence over your health, your ability to heal and, in general, your immune system. If I were asked to identify the master switch in the body most influential over your health or disease, I would say the brain stem region.

Structurally, the brain stem is located at the base of the brain. It is also the beginning of the very top of the spinal cord. The brain stem, for the most part, is contained just inside the bottom of the skull and is partly protected by the very top vertebra known as C-1, more commonly called the Atlas.

If the upper cervical spinal cord, or the brain stem, has pressure on it or is irritated because the top neck vertebra is slightly malpositioned, then the result is an altered function of an organ or a system of your body. This scenario is similar to a transformer blowing out at a neighborhood substation. A lot of houses may have a power loss. As in the neighborhood and in the body, a loss of the normal transmission of power will eventually reek havoc. Yet, in the body you may not notice it for a good while. This is so important, yet this reality that one can have malfunction before symptom is overlooked by most people, including MDs, and even a fair number of

Doctors of Chiropractic. Unfortunately, many doctors get caught up in treating symptoms, rather than getting to the cause. Remember, we desire to strike at the core of health amplification. If the cause of the problem is eliminated, the symptoms will take care of themselves.

Let me restate what *Gray's Anatomy*, the leading anatomical textbook used throughout the free world, tells us about the brain and spinal cord. Paraphrased, it tells us that *the purpose of the brain and spinal cord is to control and coordinate all the tissues, organs, and systems of the body and to adapt the organism ... you ... to the environment.* Now, that's so important, let's read it again ... The purpose of the brain and spinal cord is to control and coordinate all the tissues, organs, and systems of the body and to <u>adapt</u> the organism to the environment! So, when it's 70 degrees inside, and you walk outside and it's 30 degrees, your body automatically adapts, you don't have to even think about it. Otherwise you'd die. If there are bugs and germs in the air you are breathing, your body adapts to, and neutralizes, them. That's why Key #6 is your "<u>Master Control Key</u>"! Your brain and spinal cord will tell your body how to neutralize those substances and your body can deal with them through this miracle called life! The brain and spinal cord, running roughshod over the trillions and trillions of cells that comprise your body, directly influence the degree of life that your various parts enjoy.

Any interference to the normal functions of the nerve system and, in particular, the brain stem region can have disastrous effects on the balance of normal health within (see Figure on next page).

There is a morbid condition that occurs to the vast majority of people we've observed with chronic headaches. This con

Effects of Spinal Misalignment

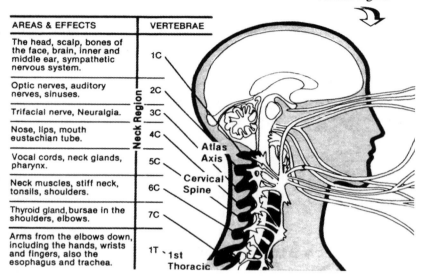

Nerves leading to various organs

AREAS & EFFECTS	VERTEBRAE
The head, scalp, bones of the face, brain, inner and middle ear, sympathetic nervous system.	1C
Optic nerves, auditory nerves, sinuses.	2C
Trifacial nerve, Neuralgia.	3C
Nose, lips, mouth eustachian tube.	4C
Vocal cords, neck glands, pharynx.	5C
Neck muscles, stiff neck, tonsils, shoulders.	6C
Thyroid gland, bursae in the shoulders, elbows.	7C
Arms from the elbows down, including the hands, wrists and fingers, also the esophagus and trachea.	1T

Neck Region

Atlas
Axis
Cervical Spine
1st Thoracic

dition can even occur initially with no outward symptoms whatsoever. It is called Atlas Neuro-Vascular Syndrome (ANVS). The Atlas is the very top vertebra of your spine. It has some very unique structural characteristics and has significant influence upon the blood supply to the brain and head. The Atlas also can effect the neurological state of the brain stem/spinal cord. Hence, the name Atlas Neuro-Vascular Syndrome. ANVS is a subclassification of a condition that most chiropractors deal with called vertebral subluxation. Now, that's an unusual term. Let's break it down. Vertebra relates to the bones of the spine. Sub-lux-ation ... the prefix "sub" means below or small. "Lux" has to do with light or life. "Ation" means a condition of. So, a <u>subluxation</u> refers to a small misalignment of the bones of the spine creating a condition of less life. Vertebral subluxation involves not just a bone pressing on nerves, but a complex relationship of vertebrae, neuro tissues, blood vessels, muscle, ligaments and other connective tissues. VS (Vertebral subluxation) can be *the* overlooked factor that is choking off Life-force, causing you, against your will and without your knowledge, to experience less "health" than your God-given birthright offers. There is really no way that you can know whether or not you have a subluxation without taking yourself to a qualified doctor of chiropractic and having your spine checked for vertebral sub-luxation. I'm a chiropractor and I don't know when my own spine is subluxated. Get yourself to a doctor who is able and dedicated to connecting your healing nerve system back to your body.

Let me give you a metaphor to make this easy to understand. There is a large artery in your body called the aorta that car-ries substantial amounts of blood from your heart to the rest of your body. If I could convince you to allow a surgeon to open you up, wrap a piece of string around your aorta, and put a knot in that string to diminish or choke down the amount of blood that could flow through your aorta, you would prob-ably agree that this situation would cause eventual problems for your body. You'd probably agree that the restriction in the flow of your blood would cause the body to become sick and even die.

This is the same thing that a subluxation does to your nerve system. A vertebral subluxation clogs the nerve system and can also affect the flow of blood. Chiropractic is that simple. We are trying to open up the Life-force.   In addition, pa-tients with chronic headache may have ANVS which com-pounds the vertebral subluxation. If the patient has not re-sponded to traditional care, it is very possible that he or she has ANVS (more on ANVS later).

But you know, *Gray's Anatomy* really didn't fully explain the big idea, either. It's not really the brain and the spinal cord that do all these wonderful acts for you, but rather the "magic" that resides in the nerve system. It's the Life-force or the innate inborn intelligence... the tiny rivulet of force that flows over the nervous system and stirs your cells into life. Let me explain. A dead human being, a corpse, has a brain and a spinal cord. But a corpse is not adapting, nor is it alive. There is no Life-force present, and that's the point. A corpse has all the physical parts necessary, but the intangible, the immeasurable force called "life" is missing. And when you allow yourself to live your life with Vertebral subluxation, unknowingly (until now), you allow yourself to live on perhaps 1/4 or 1/2 of your available power! Thus, you are setting the stage for you to experience ill health (such as headaches), regardless of the diagnosis you and your doctors have put on your condition. The flow of Life-force is **The Master Foundational Key**.

Wouldn't your body be better able to heal, to rebound and to remain fully alive without Vertebral Subluxation and other interferences to your nervous system and Life-force? The answer is ABSOLUTELY! Every aspect of your life must be stronger when the Life-force is cleared of obstructions. My job is like that of a locksmith responsible for figuring out your combination, and opening the tumblers of health without adding more chemicals to your body, without doing surgery. Let's open your channels so that the "stuff" of life can freely flow from above, down and inside out. And this locked up Life-force can be the most important and over-looked factor in your health regime.

Hippocrites, the father of medicine over 300 hundred years before the time of Christ said, "Look well to the spine for the cause of disease." You look closely to Foundational Key # 6, A Healthy Spine and Nerve System.

Now your educated mind has learned about the healthy six. **The Six Foundational Keys to Health**.

Action Step: The only way that I know to ensure that the Life-force is flowing, is to consult with a chiropractor who utilizes an approach to get and keep the nerve pathways open and clear. I'm not talking about receiving random manipulations to the spine, but rather, scientifically designed and applied adjustment/corrections.

Now, let's examine the final concept, that will weave together the final threads of this tapestry for bottom-line results. You've reviewed the 6 Foundational Keys to health amplification. I am hopeful that you are beginning to employ a portion or all of the Keys.

Now, for those with "extremely frustrating recurring" headaches, <u>regardless</u> of what you've been told and whom you've previously consulted, in the final chapter I want to introduce you to a new paradigm. From ancient times we have the story of the flight of the Phoenix. Out of the ashes flew this bird, from impossible beginnings. In our modern day, regarding your equally miraculous recovery, let's simply refer to this mindset and effort as the place ......

• Chapter Thirteen •

WHERE THE RUBBER MEETS THE ROAD

*"The road to success is always
under construction."*
-- unknown

The concept of getting one's nerve system opened up through specific spinal adjustments, allowing the body parts to work more harmoniously advancing one's wellness, has long been a central theme in chiropractic. Millions of people enjoy the many benefits of tradi-

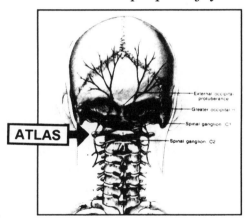

tional chiropractic. However, if you are found to have Atlas Neuro-Vascular Syndrome you may never receive the benefit from

ATLAS

traditional chiropractic (or any other traditional discipline) that you are seeking. If <u>ANVS</u> is the root cause of your headaches, you will need specific technology to reduce/remove that condition. In my opinion, this is where the "rubber meets the road" in chronic and previously non-responding headache cases.

If your health needs are being fulfilled through any health discipine or method, then I celebrate with you. I encourage you to stick with it. If, on the other hand, you have concerns particularly as they relate to chronic headache and the immune system, then you should be aware that you may have ANVS and there is another path you must investigate.

Your health problem is unique, just as you are unique. If you don't get favorable results from your general medical practitioner, you're not likely to get upset and give up on the whole medical profession. What most people do is find themselves a new doctor or a specialist and proceed from there. Not realizing that we have specialties within chiropractic, some people might give up when they are only inches away from success. Determined persistence is exactly what you must maintain for yourself regardless of how many doctors, or different types of doctors, you've consulted and in spite of what they've told you. Right now you may be discovering the technology to literally reshape your life and your future. Today nearly all doctors of chiropractic, and many progressive medical doctors, recognize that there are specialties within the profession that produce fabulous results for particular conditions. Over the years I've noticed only average success for low back disorders in our clinic, though we've consistently had huge success with neck and head cases that, in actuality, *"shouldn't have responded."* These successes have led me to dedicate more effort toward chronic headaches, and I am now specializing in the "impossible" cases.

At the Finnigan Center, in addition to our Life-force instruction, we employ a specialized procedure designed to "connect" the healing portion of the brain (the brain stem) back to the body. This system is called "Atlas Orthogonal procedures" (A.O.). A.O. is a wonderful balancing approach to healing. The A.O. technique often allows us to help certain cases, particularly headache cases who were not previously responding to traditional methods. You may decide to come to us on your own, which you are welcome to do without a doctor's referral. We will do all we can in two or three days to connect the flow of the Life-force back to your body. I personally instruct patients in protecting and amplifying the results we achieve. Then (if appropriate), we consult with referring doctors as we send our patient's back to them for

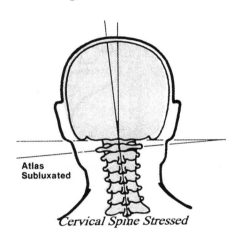

**Atlas
Subluxated**

Cervical Spine Stressed

supportive care. A.O. requires precision instrumentation, years of clinical experience, and post graduate studies. At this writing there are only about 45 doctors worldwide who are certified in Atlas Orthogonal procedures. I recently returned from Australia where I met with a group of doctors who are interested in starting this procedure "down under."

The A.O. procedure employs no forceful manipulation, but rather a precision analysis of the upper cervical spine. The actual treatment feels something like a tickling vibration below the ear and behind the

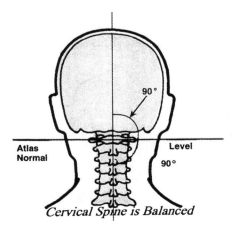

**Atlas
Normal**

90°

Level

90°

Cervical Spine is Balanced

jaw, if you feel anything at all. It is literally the introduction of a percussion wave (completely imperceptible) directed toward the Atlas vertebrae (the very top vertebrae of the spine) at a predetermined, exact vector by the Atlas Orthogonal Instrument. The instrument does not probe forward or have any excursion. Most patients who experience A.O. for the first time are surprised that such favorable results are achieved, and that no pain is associated with the procedure.

The man responsible for this Atlas Orthogonal program is Dr. Roy W. Sweat of Atlanta, Georgia. Dr. Sweat has studied the upper cervical spine and its relationship to health and disease for the better part of 40 years. Dr. Sweat has shown the tenacity and drive to invent and perfect the necessary equipment to effectively correct Atlas problems including Atlas Neuro-Vascular Syndrome. Because of his efforts his students, including myself are empowered to effectively and with precision help legions of people regain their health and once again lead productive lives. This technology is truly a breakthrough. My hat is off to you, Dr. Sweat!

In A.O., before any care is rendered, we measure exactly if, and how (in which direction), the Atlas has slid or twisted in relation to the skull, the brain stem/spinal cord and the rest of the spine. As mentioned, the Atlas is the top bone of the spine, balancing and supporting 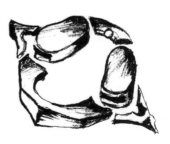 the weight of the skull. The Atlas is unusual when compared to the other spinal vertebrae, not only in its location but also its shape. The Atlas is similar to a donut, with a hole in the middle for the spinal cord to descend through. Imagine on each side of the donut a small cup to support the rockers on the base of the skull. The rockers are called condyles; they allow for movement between the skull and Atlas.

Consider the Atlas a transition point between skull and spine. It is designed to pro-

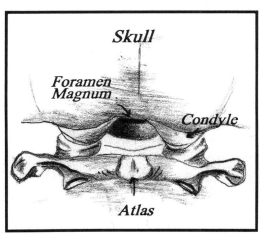

tect the brain stem and spinal cord. As with all other systems in the body, and for that matter all mechanical systems that you work with, transitional points are usually where breakdowns occur. The axle in your automobile, for instance, is not likely to break in the middle. Most problems occur at the transition between the axle and the wheel. The same is true of the Atlas region.

The bottom of the skull has a large hole in it (the Foramen Magnum) where the brain stem and spinal cord descend into the spinal column. Surrounding the hole are the two knobs, or rockers (condyles), mentioned above one on the right, and one the left of the hole. These rockers rest on the top part of the Atlas vertebra, something like a very shallow ball and socket. Meanwhile, the Atlas itself sits rather precariously on the inclined surface of the second cervical vertebrae known as the Axis.

There are two factors that are particularly unusual about the Atlas transitional area. 1) In other areas of the spine the vertebrae have an interlocking mechanism (called facets) preventing the vertebrae from twisting or subluxating too far. Unlike the rest of the spine, the Atlas has no locks; it functions much like a universal joint. There are muscles and ligaments, but they don't check the motion as effectively as the structural facets of the lower spine. In addition, the Atlas' articulating surfaces are very slippery, with a friction co-efficient of .005 (almost like ice skating). 2) An incredible amount of neurological and vascular influence over the organism (you) passing through and around the Atlas.

An unfortunate example of the importance of the Atlas area is the well-recognized actor Christopher Reeve, who portrayed *Superman* in the movies. You may recall Mr. Reeve was thrown from the horse he was riding. He landed in such a way that he broke his neck. It is sad that this wonderful person and role model became paralyzed, yet, he is fortunate to be alive considering what could have happened. The good news is he continues as a role model, only now his attention is on those with similar spinal cord injuries.

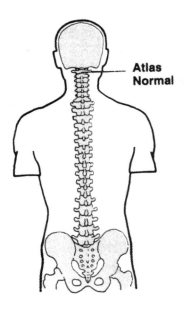

**Atlas
Normal**

Frequently, a fractured Atlas is a death sentence. Many state penal systems have learned an interesting anatomy lesson from the cattle rustlers of the old West. When a rope is looped around the top of the neck and the victim is dropped a few feet, the spinal cord is ruptured at the Atlas level. This person does not choke to death, as some people might think, his body ceases to function in short order due to neurological interruption as the Atlas is shoved into the spinal cord. This is an extreme example, and I don't intend to offend readers, but I do want to share the impact and importance of the nerve system, particularly the Atlas area. Mainly, for the vascular and neurological reasons stated above, I don't believe the Atlas should be randomly manipulated. I feel that we must deal with the Atlas in a very exact fashion, with a systematic feedback protocol to ensure progress.

The influence of the Atlas over the body is misunderstood, underestimated and hardly noticed until one has a personal experience with it. We have included a number of personal experiences in the back of the book. Medical journals are beginning to publish articles on various aspects of Atlas influence, including implications ranging from clinical depression and suicidal tendencies, to immunological disorders. You see, if the Atlas is slightly malpositioned (subluxated) then it likely will produce an alteration in the pathways of the spinal cord and/or the blood vessels passing to and from the brain. Just a slight twist of the Atlas for some people can cause a variety of symptoms, while in other people it can cause chronic headaches, low energy, insomnia, chronic neck and back pain, vertigo, or even degenerative diseases if neglected long enough.

I recently coined the phrase "Atlas Neuro-Vascular Syndrome (ANVS)" to help doctors and patients realize that this area needs to be taken seriously. ANVS is terminology that is more descriptive and accurate when dealing with particular complex cases involving the upper cervical spine. ANVS helps us realize that the Atlas can subluxate, causing a syndrome involving the neurological tissues and also causing vascular compromise. In my opinion, ANVS is one of the most insidious and morbid conditions that can occur to our body today. ANVS is so stealthy, short-circuiting the body like the hands of a clock you are probably unaware of its progession until the condition has a powerful grip. Few people, including a small handful of doctors, recognize the progressive yet relentless death grip ANVS often has on its victims. Therefore, most people are given prescriptions for months and even years in an attempt to only treat the symptoms. Drugs can never correct the underlying cause of ANVS.

The chronic headache patient who has invested precious time and money into his or her problem, with no solid results, must be examined for ANVS.

By combining the preceding Life-force principles with our Atlas procedure, we have created a new paradigm for healing the mind and body. I am hopeful that by truly embracing the Life-force Foundational Keys that you have learned in this book your personal health will soar. As mentioned, some of us only need to turn one or two keys and the body responds. If, however, you are not observing the break-throughs that you hoped for, if traditional methods haven't moved you on top, then perhaps you have ANVS in addition to the other Foundational Keys that need to be engaged.

I would like to take a couple of paragraphs to encourage the readers who are feeling discouraged, those who feel like they've tried everything and they're still sick and tired ... don't quit now!

You need to be aware of some of the results our patients have received. You might consider them nothing short of miraculous. But you may not care about the recoveries others have experienced- you want to know if the Life-force/Atlas program will work for you. First, apply to your life, everything we've written about and turn "on" as many of the keys as you possibly can.

After working in these areas, I'm confident that 80 persent or more of you r eading this book will respond favorably without consulting me.

If, however, you don't feel you've gotten as far as you should, and you're committed to getting results, then I want to hear from you.

Our Life-force/Atlas system is a specialized program. It is a two-and-one-half day intensive program designed to get results for the very tough cases. After you've completed the program I'll send you back to your doctor for follow up and support.

The impossible cases are the ones I love! Helping people who have tried traditional approaches, that simply haven't worked is what I live for. Amazingly, after our procedure, many of these patients are able to return to their previous treatment programs, and begin to respond favorably and resume their lives.

If you fall into this category as non-responsive to traditional methods, yet you are still committed to getting your chronic headache problem resolved, then perhaps I can help. *I will stand, or fall, on your results.* You have nothing to risk except travel costs and some time. **We will accept all financial risk for your care** ... and if you don't receive a favorable response *immediately* with our Life-force/Atlas program, then you don't pay for any treatment cost, only a modest fee for exam and X-ray. We part as friends. What could be more fair than that?

I am very confident that this technology will produce results. If you are serious about changing this part of your life, then we are willing to offer a complimentary consultation so you can investigate without any expense. For our "out-of-town guests" we do a lot of consultations over the phone as a first step. Then, if we agree to work together, we will completely stand behind our results. I know of no other health restoration program willing to provide such a generous opportunity. Come visit our office in beautiful Olympia, Washington. Plan on a two-and-a-half-day stay (minimum— stay longer if you wish to enjoy our clean air and breathtaking scenery) here in the Puget Sound area. You'll have time to visit the Cascade Mountains or take in the sights of Seattle. During your restful visit to our community, we will give you one-on-one attention to see that you get the correction you so desperately want and need.

If you are traveling from out of the area, plan to arrive at our office at or before 5 P.M. on a Monday. You will attend a brief discussion of the Life-force principles (this is required for new patients wishing to take advantage of our no-risk opportunity), followed by an examination.

The next morning (Tuesday), we will begin working with you. By noon, you'll know if we are on the right track ... or not. You will be given the opportunity to continue on with the program and "go for it," or request and receive a full refund of your deposit and we'll part as friends.

After lunch, if you decide to go forward with the program, we will re-check the progress you're making, do some fine-tuning, if necessary, and give you information that will enhance the long-term benefits you'll receive from the treatment. We will monitor and fine-tune your Life-force again late Tuesday and again on Wednesday morning.

You'll be on your way home by noon on Wednesday, absolutely thrilled and, perhaps, for the first time in years, confident and excited about your future ... or you will have left Tuesday owing nothing!

It has never been easier to discover a healing program that will end your pain and suffering once and for all. Because you may be traveling hundreds of miles or more to consult with me, I want to make sure that you completely understand I have nothing to gain unless you are absolutely thrilled with your care. This is why the telephone consultation is often a good first step. If you decide to visit us be sure to request information on the "fly for free" program

FOUNDATIONAL KEY ACTION LIST

1. *Start breathing!* Feed those cells oxygen and pump that lymph.

2. *Food and water ...*
   A.   Make sure your water is pure, please don't take it for granted.
   B.   Start eating larger percentages of uncooked enzymatically alive foods. Five or more servings of raw fruits and vegetables *every day* or suitable supplements (see appendix for product information).
   C.   Try to combine your meals correctly -- more often.

3. *Exercise* ... Get some form of frequent fun activity.   Move those muscles, activate the heart, pump that lymph. There is a law in physiology ... "What you don't use ... you lose."

4. *Sleep ...* What a pleasure. One third of your life ... enjoy it on your back or side. Please use a moderate-sized pillow.

5. *Positive Mental Attitude* ... There are hundreds of good books on this subject. Have you read one lately? The audio cassette player in my car turns travel time into a classroom. Why listen to the news when you can pump your brain with positive, productive and resourceful thoughts?

6. **The Master Key:** the most overlooked, least understood, aspect of health and recovery. How can an eight cylinder automobile engine function on four spark plugs? People who are living with ANVS are a lot like an automobile trying to make it up "life's hills" on three or four cylinders. You really don't have a chance. However, when the Atlas is balanced and reconnected, the power is turned back on, and you are firing on all cylinders! At that moment all of the other five **Foundational Keys** are more cooperative. Secondary treatment plans work better. The immune system is advanced. Simply ...You're more alive with the Life-force fully lit. And, oh yes, your long-standing head-aches amazingly dissolve.

I'd like to close this, my first book, with an *Irish Blessing* my wife framed for me — it hangs in my study ...

"May the road rise up to meet you. May the wind always be at your back. May the sun shine warm on your face, the rains fall soft upon your fields, and, until we meet again.... may God hold you softly in the palm of his hand."

So long for now, and may God bless you.

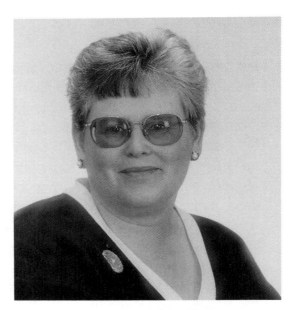

Dolly Kelly

• Testimonials •

I had been suffering with continuous severe headaches for years. I can safely say that the headaches had altered my views on life, and my personality. The pain was all over my head, and at times it was necessary for me to confine myself to bed from the accompanying nausea.

Medications would temporarily lessen the pain but never completely removed it, and besides the pills were only treating the symptom, not the cause. I have never received any satisfaction for this problem from any medical doctor.

When I first met Dr. Finnigan, I found him to be genuinely concerned, friendly, and very informative. What really is unusual was his unique approach to my problem. His equipment, and techniques provided results superior to my expectation, and there has been no pain whatsoever with any treatment, in fact it is kind of fun to go to his office.

In addition to my headache problems being resolved, I have more energy, and I can think better! But the most interesting phenomena that I've noticed since having my correction is that I am now remembering the dreams that I have at night. As far as I was concerned I hadn't had dreams for ten years or more!

If you are suffering from chronic headaches and all that goes with them, and if you've tried everything else like I had, then you've got nothing to lose. This is different, give his office a call.

Dolly Kelly

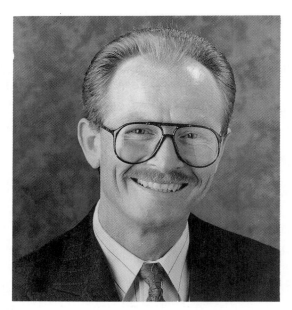

Mark Van Hemert DC DACS

Dear Dr. Finnigan:

It has been a pleasure to be associated with you and your upper cervical specific technique during the past several years. During my years of practice, I have noted the wonderful response that patients have with chiropractic care. However, I have also noted that some of my cervical cases were unresponsive to my particular technique. For years I had wished that there was an upper cervical specialist that I could refer to. Then, about four years ago, I learned that you were practicing "A.O." I decided to refer an unresponsive patient to your clinic. The patients response was miraculous. She immediately noticed a reduction in her cervical pain and unrelenting headache. I have since referred all my unresponsive cervical patients to you for evaluation and care. My patients are not only excited about the response that they receive from your procedures, but they have also commented about the warmth of your staff and yourself.

My patients also have a higher opinion of my diagnostic skill, if I am able to make a referral that results in the reduction of their pain. I have often wondered why many doctors of chiropractic, when their particular approach is not effective for an individual's problem, will refer the patient to a medical doctor instead of a chiropractic specialist. It only makes sense to refer within the profession, if the diagnosis is VSC of the spine.

Keep up the excellent work Jeff, and as BJ said, "Chiropractic must be specific or it is nothing at all."

                        Sincerely,
                        Mark Van Hemert DC DACS

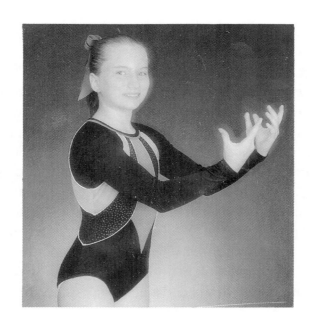

Sarah Lebow

Our daughter, Sarah, is in competitive gymnastics. She started having significant reoccurring headaches nearly every day, about three years ago. The cause of the headaches seem to stem from two accidents. First, an automobile accident, later, and more obvious, was a fall while roller skating. As the headaches continued over time, they became more intense. The condition began to wear on her, and certainly affected her athletic performance.

We consulted a number of physicians. They recommended Tylenol, and other over-the-counter medications. If they helped at all, the headaches would return at full force after the drug wore off. We also had her eyes checked all to no avail.

One of Sarah's gymnastic team mate's mother told us about, and recommended Dr. Finnigan's special approach. We had our doubts, but had nothing to lose.

When we went to Dr. Finnigan's office, we found the staff very helpful and friendly. The results were immediate and profound. After the first visit, Sarah went several days without any headache whatsoever! Now, over a year and one half later, it's a rare occasion that she mentions any headache pain. If she does have one, the intensity is far less than before. We're certain that this program has made a 100% improvement in Sarah's life.

We're happy to share Sarah's story because some people might think children can't have debilitating headaches. Well, they can. We have living proof. And this program has produced results, safely and comfortably, while everything else simply treated the symptoms.

Angela and Donald Lebow

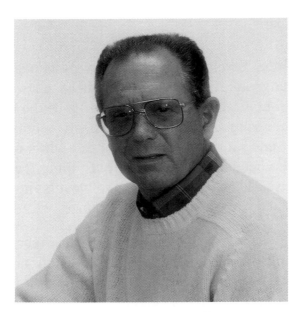

Tom Harpel

In a 1979 industrial accident I did some damage to my back and neck while working in the long shore industry. I spent the next couple years with doctors and physical therapists. I took drugs such as Percocet and Darvon with only minimal relief. I was unable to resume my normal activities, both at home and at work, without significant pain.

Frequent headaches would cause so much pain that I'd be sick to the point that it would create sessions of vomiting. And that situation was creating stress at home with the family. I also had back pain.

It was just chance (or providential intervention) that I found myself in Dr. Finnigan's office. At first I wasn't sure if I was doing the right thing, but I hadn't gotten results elsewhere.

He took x-rays, and spent a great deal of time explaining how he thought he would be able to help, he also explained what would be my responsibilities. Then I learned how the Atlas was causing a majority of my problems.

Within a short period of time I was feeling better, however in the beginning he did meet me at his office at 3 A.M. a couple times when I had a sick headache. He's told me that I was one of his toughest patients ever, yet in spite of that we've become friends.

I've referred a number of people to Dr. Jeff, and I encourage you to come have a look if you've not gotten the results, and correction that you desire.

Tom Harpel

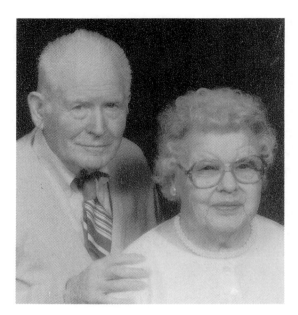

Orvis C. Owens

I went to Dr. Finnigan some years ago for a back condition that he promptly took care of. I had no further need of his services for about five years. This time he detected something wrong in the top of my neck even though my complaint again was down low. He worked on me a few times, and my back began to improve. But, what really surprised and astonished my wife and I was the severe vertigo (dizziness) that I have continually suffered with since 1950 (45 years!) is totally gone!

The vertigo is so bad sometimes that it would make me sick to my stomach. I'd have to hold onto someone or something in order not to fall down. I always have to avoid making quick motions.

I have taken Arliden and more recently Mecclizine everyday to "manage" my vertigo. These drugs have provided some relief, but I always still had the problem, and who knows what side effects can come from these drugs.

I had no expectations that Dr. Finnigan's approach could erase a 45 year case of vertigo. I thought I would spend the rest of my life fighting my dizziness. I want to encourage anyone who has suffered with ongoing headaches or vertigo to give Dr. Finnigan a call ... especially if you've been told you'll have to live with your problem. You have absolutely nothing to lose except your pain.

Orvis C. Owens

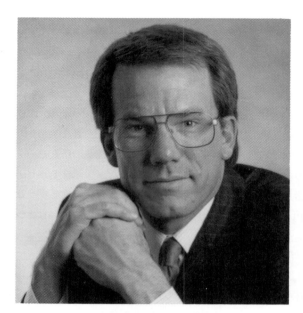

Dr. Richard Benson

As a practicing doctor of chiropractic for 18 years, I have a healthy respect for the power in life and the ability of the body to heal and maintain itself healthfully. However, there are situations (such as chronic headaches) that are given up for hopeless. There is a technology for the correction of these "hopeless" cases ... and that technology resides in Dr. Finnigan's office. I've personally seen him at work, and had my life enhanced through his methods. Anyone with chronic headaches (particularly if you've been told you'll have to live with the problem), should seriously consider a short stay with Dr. Jeff. I don't have headaches, but I personally travel 300 miles to his office a couple times per year to make sure my Life-force is not interfered with.

Dr. Richard Benson

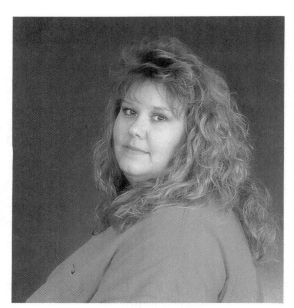

Cody Hobson

I had been suffering from frequent headaches for about five years. The computer work that I was required to do contributed to continual neck and upper back pain. By late morning I would have a "stress headache" that I would take home nearly every work day.

My sister referred me to Dr. Finnigan, and when I finally got myself to the office, I found a warm atmosphere, and a doctor who was interested not just in treating the symptoms, but, rather, correcting the cause. Immediately after my first painless Atlas adjustment, my headaches began to clear. The upper back and neck have improved, too!

But, the <u>really</u> surprising thing is about three years ago I was diagnosed with Asthma. The winter before coming to Dr. Finnigan I had over THREE WEEKS of time loss from work and I felt terrible all of the time. But now I feel great! I have taken <u>no</u> asthma medication, nor inhalers for over two years! And my headaches are a thing of the past.

I am certain my immune system is stronger than before. I have been around people who are ill all year (particularly winters) and now I stay well. I attribute my healthier immune system to the same procedure that corrected my headaches.

Don't let distance or finance prevent you from at least investigating this program. Dr. Finnigan is as close as your phone. I don't have any insurance coverage for this, but I've found that it is affordable. This has been a great investment. My health is a nonrenewable asset. Without your health you've got nothing! If you have chronic headaches, this program was designed for you.

Cody Hobson

Information Card

For information on available dates, investment, and travel arrangements for Dr. Finnigan's Life-force A.O. programs call 1(360) 459-7800, 9:30 a.m. to 5 p.m. (Pacific time), and our staff will answer your questions. If calling after hours, leave your name and number and we'll return your call, or write to us at: 1307 Violet S.E., Olympia, Washington 98503.

The program typically begins Monday afternoon by 5 p.m. and ends Wednesday by noon. We have hotels of various price ranges near by. Our center is located in Olympia, Washington, one hour south of Sea Tac Airport, or 90 miles north of the Portland, Oregon airport, on Interstate 5.

— over —

Product Information

Dr. Finnigan mentioned two products which are available for purchase. Counter-top water filtration systems from National Safety Associates, which are effective and simple to use, have a price range of around $179, plus appropriate tax and shipping directly to your home.

— over —

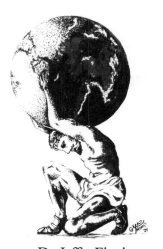

Life-force Atlas Orthogonal Programs

1307 Violet S.E.

Olympia, Washington 98503

(360) 459-7800

Product Information

The nutritional product is a "whole food" rather than a fragmented vitamin or mineral. It is called Juice Plus+, and provides a much wider variety of naturally-occurring vitamins and minerals from a wide variety of sources. It also provides the phytochemicals, antioxidants, active enzymes, chlorophyll, and other nutrients — and ever the fiber — from the fresh, raw fruits and vegetables it's made from. Juice Plus+ comes in a capsule form. Take two fruit capsules with water or juice in the morning, and two vegetable capsules with dinner. Juice Plus+ is a convenient and economical way to enhance your nutritional needs, For about $1.40 per day, you'll get the nutritional benefits of several pounds of produce. One carton of Juice Plus+ will provide the recommended trial period of four months. That's normally $179 plus shipping and tax.

Your Doctor

If you have purchased this book from your doctor, chances are good he or she is also one of the select few Atlas Orthogonists mentioned in the preceding pages.

I have asked your doctor to stamp their name below so that as you share this information with your family and friends they too will have access to these benefits.